The Cortisol Connection

WHY STRESS MAKES YOU FAT AND RUINS YOUR HEALTH — AND WHAT YOU CAN DO ABOUT IT

. . . .

Shawn M. Talbott, Ph.D.

Foreword by William J. Kraemer, Ph.D.

Hunter House
PUBLISHERS

Hunter House Inc., Publishers
PO Box 2914
Alameda CA 94501-0914

Library of Congress Cataloging-in-Publication Data

Talbott, Shawn M.
The cortisol connection : why stress makes you fat and ruins your health -- and what you can do about it / Shawn M. Talbott.-- 1st ed.
p. cm.
Includes bibliographical references and index.
ISBN 0-89793-392-3 (cl) -- ISBN 0-89793-391-5 (pb)
1. Stress management. 2. Stress (Physiology). 3. Hydrocortisone--Physiological effect. 4. Health. 5. Obesity. I. Title.

RA785 .T35 2002
155.9'042--dc21   2002068686

Project Credits

Cover Design: Jil Weil Design
Book Production: Hunter House, Buchman Bookworks
Developmental and Copy Editor: Kelley Blewster
Proofreader: Rachel E. Bernstein
Indexer: Nancy D. Petersen
Acquisitions Editor: Jeanne Brondino
Editor: Alexandra Mummery
Editorial Assistance: Claire Reilly-Shapiro
Sales & Marketing Coordinator: JoAnne Retzlaff
Publicity Coordinator: Earlita K. Chenault
Customer Service Manager: Christina Sverdrup
Order Fulfillment: Lakdhon Lama
Administrator: Theresa Nelson
Computer Support: Peter Eichelberger
Publisher: Kiran S. Rana

Printed and Bound by Transcontinental Printing, Canada

9 8 7   First Edition   04 05 06

Contents

Foreword

The adrenal hormone "cortisol" has essentially become how "stress" is defined. Stress and cortisol have been the topic of intense interest in both the scientific and lay press for over fifty years. From the pioneering laboratory work of Dr. Hans Selye, a Canadian endocrinologist who first coined stress as a "general adaptation syndrome" to more current views of stress as a specific phenomenon, cortisol has played a key role in stress's negative effects. Cortisol plays a wide variety of physiological roles in the body and when stress produces excessive levels, problems result. In his book *The Cortisol Connection: Why Stress Makes You Fat and Ruins Your Health—and What You Can Do about It*, Dr. Talbott brings the reader up to date and into the arena of stress physiology and nutrition. Dr. Talbott provides important new insights into the physiology of stress, management techniques, and the many new and innovative methods that can be used to combat stress with nutrition. The text is well written and easy to understand. It is engaging in its presentation and is an enjoyable read. Dr. Talbott brings the needed scientific credibility to this book by drawing on his extensive experience and understanding of nutrition and stress physiology. The book provides one of the first informative texts for both the lay public and medical professionals. This book is important to us all, as each of us face a host of stresses in our everyday lives that can potentially increase cortisol and affect our health. The importance of nutrition, and the role certain nutritional supplements can play in helping to combat stress and the negative effects of excessive cortisol responses, is one of the real hallmarks of Dr. Talbott's work. Thus, the book provides a host of valuable information and practical ideas while being carefully crafted to give the reader the needed understanding and insights to take control of one's lifestyle to eliminate the negative effects that too much cortisol can have in the body. I believe this book is a must read for anyone interested in improving one's health and better coping with the stresses of life through optimal nutrition.

— William J. Kraemer, Ph.D.
    Professor of Kinesiology, Physiology, and Neurobiology
    The University of Connecticut

Acknowledgments

In writing *The Cortisol Connection*, I have consulted the scientific work of hundreds of researchers and medical professionals, but in particular, the experiments of the following scientists were especially helpful: Robert Sapolsky, Ph.D., at Stanford University; George Chrousos, M.D., at the National Institutes of Health; Pamela Peeke, M.D., M.P.H., at the University of Maryland School of Medicine; Per Bjorntorp, M.D., Ph.D., at the University of Goteborg in Sweden; Susan Barr, Ph.D., at the University of British Columbia; and Elissa Epel, Ph.D., at the University of California at San Francisco.

The Cortisol Connection would not have been possible without the invaluable advice and guidance of my friends and colleagues Carsten Smidt, Ph.D., Win Duersch, Ph.D., Jeffrey Zidichouski, Ph.D., and Bill Kraemer, Ph.D.—each of whom remained an "open-minded skeptic" to help guide and refine the development of the underlying concept of the book and recommendations for cortisol control. All of the articles from Chinese journals cited in the References were summarized and/or translated for me by two colleagues: D. C. Zhang, based in Shanghai, China, and J. S. Zhu, based in Beijing, China.

I would also like to acknowledge the foresight of the editors at Hunter House Publishers, most notably Jeanne Brondino, for grasping the significant public-health benefit of bringing the concept of cortisol control to publication as quickly as possible.

In putting together this book, I was often at risk for not following my own advice about controlling my cortisol levels. Despite knowing quite clearly that depriving myself of sleep or drinking too much coffee or skipping a workout might increase my short-term productivity (by helping me get more pages written), I also knew that these practices would certainly increase my cortisol levels and do "bad things" to me in the long run. Luckily, added reinforcement and willpower to do the right thing and follow my own advice was ever present in the form of my loving wife and best friend, Julie Talbott. Always there to remind me to "take your own advice!" (including the exclamation point), Julie provides the same balance to my work that she has forever provided to our relationship and to my life—and for that I dedicate this book to her.

IMPORTANT NOTE

The material in this book is intended to provide a review of information regarding the effects on health of stress and cortisol. Every effort has been made to provide accurate and dependable information. The contents of the book have been compiled through professional research and in consultation with medical professionals. However, scientists and health-care professionals often have differing opinions about the rapid advancements in nutrition and supplement science. It is important to appreciate the fact that advances in medical and scientific research are made very quickly, so some of the information in this book may become outdated.

Therefore, the publisher, authors, and editors, and the professionals quoted in the book cannot be held responsible for any error, omission, or dated material. The authors, editors, and publisher assume no responsibility for any outcome of applying the information in this book in a program of self-care or under the care of a licensed practitioner. If you have questions concerning your nutrition or diet, or about the application of the information described in this book, consult a qualified health-care professional.

Preface

Got stress? Of *course* you do! That's strike one.

How about sleep—do you get at least eight solid hours of restful sleep every night? No? Strike two.

What about your diet—are you among the millions of people who are actively dieting or concerned about what you eat? Yes? Strike three.

With three strikes, you are hereby officially welcomed as a card-carrying member of the Cortisol Club—and it's killing you.

Like virtually every other student of the life sciences, I first learned about cortisol (the primary stress hormone) many years ago in Biology 101. There, we all learned that cortisol was part of the famous "fight-or-flight" reaction to stress—a reaction that occurs much the same way in monkeys and zebras and gazelles as it does in you and me. You probably know how it goes: the lion jumps out of the bushes; the zebra gets scared, mounts a hormonal stress response, and runs away; end of stress response. Like most students (maybe yourself included), I also learned that while stress rapidly increases cortisol levels, removing the stress tends to bring those elevated levels back down to normal. Little did we know or appreciate back then, however, that the many forms of modern stress we all experience on a daily basis (jobs, kids, traffic, bills, etc.) cause the very same elevation in our cortisol levels—but removing those stressors is not an option for most of us. As a result, these chronic stressors cause our cortisol levels to stay high and lead us down the road to poor health.

Perhaps the biggest problem with chronic stress and elevated cortisol levels is the fact that the initial effects are so subtle—a few extra pounds of weight, a slight reduction in energy levels, a modest drop in sex drive, a bit of trouble with memory—that we simply brush them off as "normal" aspects of aging. However, as *The Cortisol Connection: Why Stress Makes You Fat and Ruins Your Health—and What You Can Do about It* will show, these effects are actually the earliest signs of obesity, diabetes, impotence, dementia, heart disease, cancer, and many related conditions. Indeed, cortisol is emerging as a key factor in the very process we all recognize as "aging."

Science is often portrayed as occurring in "Eureka!" moments of breakthrough thinking by brilliant minds. While the "Eureka!" scenes might look good in Hollywood films, more often than not the really important concepts in science and medicine are the result of the relentless and painstaking work of many researchers conducted over many years. Such is the case with the concepts outlined in *The Cortisol Connection*. In this regard, I am neither a specialized stress physiologist nor an endocrinologist, but a broadly trained nutritionist who is bringing together the published research of many excellent scientists. Additionally, in the mid-1990s, some of my own laboratory work showed that rats exposed to the "stress" of a weight-loss diet experienced elevated cortisol levels and reduced bone strength—suggesting that dieting and stress could increase the risk of osteoporosis. Decades prior to my own research, however, pioneers in stress research, including the "father" of stress physiology, Hans Selye, had already shown that chronic stress interferes with normal metabolism in a variety of ways. In his series of experiments, Dr. Selye showed that stress caused animals to develop ulcers, get sick, and die earlier than their nonstressed counterparts. Bad stuff.

Unfortunately, even though researchers and medical professionals have *suspected* a similar connection between human stress and our risk of certain diseases since Selye's earliest work, it has been difficult to clearly *show* this relationship in a clinical study. As a result, many of us have tended to think of stress as a normal part of life that we simply have to deal with as well as we can. In the last four or five years, however, we have seen a tremendous amount of research into the effects of stress on long-term health. During that same period, and especially within the past year or so, several lines of evidence have converged to solidify the concept that stress makes us fat (because of cortisol), thins our bones (because of cortisol), shrinks our brains (because of cortisol), suppresses our immune system (because of cortisol), saps our energy levels (because of cortisol), and kills our sex drive (because of cortisol). Bad news, to be sure, but the good news is that you can do something about it, and this is where *The Cortisol Connection* can help. Through an easy-to-follow program—called SENSE—you can learn how to incorporate stress management, exercise, nutrition, and dietary supplements into a realistic (that is, very doable) approach to controlling cortisol levels.

I feel very strongly—in fact, I am *certain*—that once you understand the relationship between modern stressors, your cortisol level, and its effects on your long-term health, you will be motivated to do something about getting your cortisol levels under control.

But first, let's see if you qualify for the program: Let's check your exposure to stress.

Gauging Your Exposure to Stress

Unless you are fully attuned to listening to your body, as an elite athlete may be accustomed to doing, it can be very difficult to read the telltale signs associated with stress-induced health problems, such as those described in the preceding few paragraphs. Therefore, it may be helpful to gauge your overall exposure to stress using the simple questionnaire presented below, which I call the Stress Self-Test. This series of questions can help you decide whether your body may be exposed to excessive cortisol levels on a regular basis.

Stress Self-Test

Directions

- For each question, write your score in the corresponding column.
- For each answer of Never/No, give yourself zero (0) points.
- For each answer of Occasionally, give yourself one (1) point.
- For each answer of Frequently/Yes, give yourself two (2) points.
- Add the numbers to obtain your total score.
- Your total score indicates your Cortisol Index.

Question   Never *or* No: 0 points / Occasionally: 1 point / Frequently *or* Yes: 2 points

How often do you experience stressful situations? _____

How often do you feel tired or fatigued for no apparent reason? _____

How often do you get less than eight hours of sleep? _____

How often do you feel anxious or depressed? _____

How often do you feel angry or aggressive? _____

How often do you feel self-conscious or inadequate? _____

How often do you feel overwhelmed or confused? _____

How often is your sex drive lower than you would like it to be? _____

Do you tend to gain weight easily? _____

Are you currently dieting? _____

How often have you attempted to control your body weight? _____

How often do you pay close attention to the foods you eat? _____

How often do you crave carbohydrates (sweets and/or breads)? _____

How often do you experience difficulty with memory or concentration? _____

How often do you experience tension headaches or muscle tightness
in your neck, shoulders, or jaw? _____

How often do you experience digestive problems such as gas,
bloating, ulcers, heartburn, constipation, or diarrhea? _____

How often do you get sick, catch colds/flu? _____

Do you have high cholesterol (greater than 200 mg/dl)? _____

Do you have high blood sugar (greater than 100 mg/dl)? _____

Do you have high blood pressure (greater than 140/90 mm/Hg)? _____

Score (add all numbers together) ____ *points*

Cortisol Index

Total Score	Stress Level	Comments
0–5 points	**Relaxed Jack:** Low risk, no worries	You are cool as a cucumber and have either a very low level of stress or a tremendous ability to deal effectively with incoming stressors.
6–10 points	**Strained Jane:** Moderate risk	You *may be* suffering from an overactive stress response and chronically elevated levels of cortisol and should incorporate antistress strategies into your lifestyle whenever possible—but don't stress out about it!
Greater than 10 points	**Stressed Jess:** High risk	You are *almost definitely* suffering from an overactive stress response and chronically elevated levels of cortisol—and you need to take immediate steps to regain control.

Are you a Stressed Jess? These days, who among us isn't? Consider the fact that virtually anybody who experiences stress on a regular basis, gets less than eight hours of sleep each night, or is either dieting or concerned about what they eat is on the fast track to elevated cortisol levels.

This is not to say that the Stressed Jesses among us are going to keel over tomorrow from cortisol overexposure—nor does it mean that the rare Relaxed Jacks in the world will necessarily live to a ripe old age. What is does mean is that each of us can benefit from targeted cortisol control. Sometimes your cortisol control regimen needs to be more aggressive (such as during times of particularly high stress), while at other times you'll have less stress in your life and you can let your attention to cortisol control wander a bit (such as during your vacation to Tahiti).

The bottom line is that living in the twenty-first century brings with it a certain amount of unavoidable stress—and with that stress comes elevated cortisol levels. It is how we deal with that stress and what we do to control those cortisol levels that make the difference when it comes to our long-term health. So keep reading. Whatever your score on the Stress Self-Test, *The Cortisol Connection: Why Stress Makes You Fat and Ruins Your Health—and What You Can Do about It* was written for you.

CHAPTER 1

Stress and Your Health: The Type C Personality

There you are, a zebra strolling across the African savanna. You're minding your own business, maybe looking for some tender young grasses to satisfy your appetite, when suddenly A LION COMES CHARGING TOWARD YOU FROM THE BUSHES! This is the classic scenario used to describe the stress response—otherwise known as the "fight-or-flight" response. In reaction to that charging lion, your body quickly paces itself through a series of neurological, biochemical, hormonal, and physiological actions—each of which is designed to help you avoid that lion (run away) and survive for another day.

In the case of the zebra, the stress response runs its complete course, from start to finish, in a relatively short period of time (Figure 1.1). The stress occurs (the charging lion), which causes the zebra's brain and hormone system to release a series of stress hormones (the stress response), which enables it to fight off the lion or run away from it (the fight-or-flight response). After getting away from the lion, the zebra's stress hormones return to normal—end of story.

Unfortunately, we humans aren't so lucky. The vast majority of our daily stressors come from things that are much scarier (or

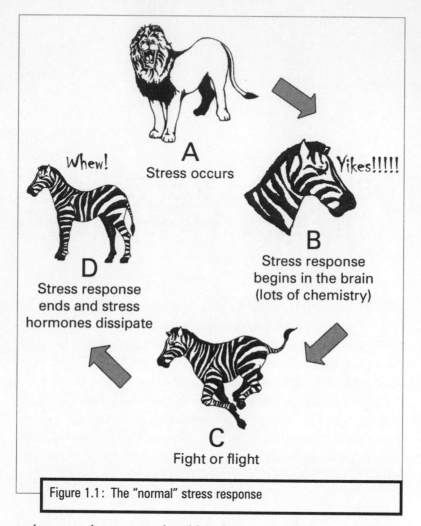

Figure 1.1: The "normal" stress response

at least much more predictable) than vicious lions—things like monthly mortgage payments, credit card bills, project deadlines, traffic jams, family commitments.... The list goes on and on. The major problem with our modern-day stressors is that they are less easy to escape from than the charging lion. The things that cause us stress today are difficult to fight off and impossible to run away from—and they also seem to keep coming back again and again. This unfortunate situation puts us in the position of being stuck midway through the normal stress response, where stress hormones are chronically elevated (Figure 1.2).

In the scenario depicted in Figure 1.2, our modern, fast-paced, high-stress lifestyles cause us to become stuck between steps B and C, creating what can be referred to as the "Type C" personality: a victim of chronic stress and elevated cortisol (hence the "C"). You have probably heard of the "Type A" and "Type B" personalities: Type A's are stereotyped as high-strung stress monsters, and Type B's are cast as laid-back folks who always roll with the

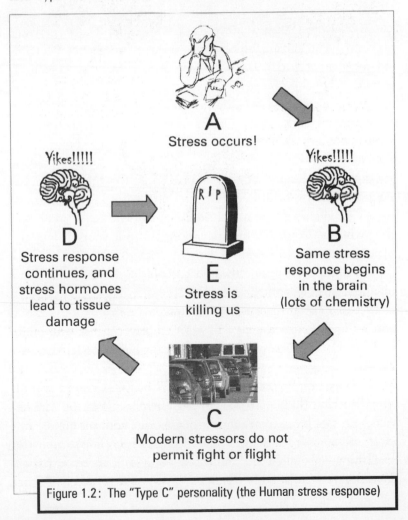

Figure 1.2: The "Type C" personality (the Human stress response)

punches. It may be obvious to you that nobody is either a "pure" Type A or Type B personality, but rather, we are all a blend of the two—some with a bit more "A" and others with a bit more "B" thrown in.

Unfortunately, we are *all* vulnerable to chronic stress and can become a Type C personality if we aren't careful to control either our *exposure* to stress or the way in which our bodies *respond* to stress. The "C" in the Type C designation also refers to the primary stress hormone—cortisol—which is elevated during periods of high stress. When we encounter something (anything) that causes us to feel stress, our cortisol levels go up. If we experience stressful events on a regular basis, and we are unable to effectively rid ourselves of the stressor, then our cortisol levels stay constantly elevated above normal levels.

Yes, you may say, bills, traffic, and the demands of work and family are all things that cause us to worry and to feel stress, but they're not exactly as life-threatening as a hungry lion bearing down on you—or are they? In cases of *acute* stress—someone sneaking up behind you and shouting "BOO!"—there are probably no long-term health consequences. In cases of *chronic* stress, however, when you ruminate, obsess, and continually mull over the "what if's" of a stressful situation, you put yourself into the Type C condition of having chronically elevated cortisol levels.

Over the long term, elevated cortisol levels can be as detrimental to overall health as elevated cholesterol is for heart disease or excessive blood sugar is for diabetes. Aside from that, elevated cortisol levels make you fat, kill your sex drive, shrink your brain, squelch your immune system, and generally make you feel terrible. So what to do?

Luckily, you have lots of choices. The easiest choice of all is to do nothing (like most people) and let chronic stress and elevated cortisol levels slowly break down your bodily defenses and increase your risk for disease. The more difficult choices are to do something—about either your stress level, the way you handle stress, or how your body responds to stressful situations. There have been at least a gazillion self-help books and empowering seminars on the general topic of "stress management," so you'll get none of that here (or at least very little). Suffice it to say that stress is a "bad thing" and stress management is a "good thing"— but because of the complexities of the topics of psychological and emotional coping, developing supportive relationships, and finding your inner self, this book will stick to some of the more concrete and practical approaches to dealing with stress: diet, exercise, and supplements.

Before we get too far into a discussion of what you can do about getting a handle on your chronic stress and elevated cortisol levels, let's talk briefly about what stress is and how it relates to your cortisol levels and overall health profile.

WHAT IS STRESS?

It's not as if you've never experienced stress. Each of us encounters stress in one form or another on a daily basis—in fact, we encounter stress multiple times during every day of our lives. Even more important, however, than the actual *things* that cause us to experience stress is our body's ability to *cope* with that stress. We're going to talk about the physiological and biochemical responses of your body to the things we identify as "stress"—and how you can customize your own approach to dealing with these internal chemical cascades.

Let's start off with a tidy definition of *stress*. For our purposes we'll define it as "what you feel when life's demands exceed your ability to meet those demands." With that said, it is important to acknowledge that everybody has a different capacity to effectively cope with stress and, thus, to "perform" when stress is encountered. Even those rare individuals who have a high tolerance for accommodating stressful situations ultimately have a breaking point—add enough total stress to *anybody* and performance suffers.

Many of the top stress researchers in the world have made the interesting distinction between the type of stressors that are faced by our cousins in the animal kingdom (short-term or *acute* stressors) and the kind with which we humans are routinely faced (longer-term and repeated *chronic* stressors). To compound our problems as "higher" animals, we are plagued not only by physical stressors but also by psychological and social stressors. Some of those psychological stressors are quite real (like your monthly rent or mortgage payment), while others are purely imaginary (like the stressful encounters that you *imagine* you might have with your boss, coworkers, kids, or others). How do you like that? Not only has our large, complex, and supposedly "advanced" brain developed the capacity to get us *out* of a whole lot of stressful situations, but it has also developed the capacity to actually *create* stressful situations where none existed before.

Robert Sapolsky, author of perhaps the best (and most readable) book on the subject of stress physiology, *Why Zebras Don't Get Ulcers* (W.H. Freeman and Company, 1998), uses the whimsical examples of zebras being stressed out by lions and baboons being stressed out by each other to illustrate the fact that short-term (acute) periods of stress are vital to survival (at least from the zebra's perspective). From his many examples, we come to learn that whereas acute periods of stress are necessary, a chronically elevated stress response is detrimental to long-term health in a variety of ways. Following the lead of Dr. Sapolsky and virtually every physiology professor who teaches about the fight-or-flight response, this book will also employ numerous examples of zebras, monkeys, and baboons to illustrate concepts related to stress physiology.

HUMANS ARE NOT ZEBRAS

Here's a vitally important point that we will come back to again and again: Human beings were simply *not* meant to carry around constant disturbances in our stress response (chronic stress); we were built to respond to stress quickly and then to have those stress hormones dissipate immediately (acute stress). When our bodies are exposed to wave after wave of stress (from our modern lifestyles), they begin to break down.

Animals don't normally harbor chronic stress the way humans do, but when they do (during stress experiments, starvation, injury, etc.) they get sick just like humans. In study after study, it quickly becomes obvious that the actual stress response, while acting as our friend in certain situations, turns against us when "everyday" events are perceived by the body as "stressful" events. Over time, stress-related diseases result from either an over-exaggerated stress response (too much response to what should have been a small stressor) or an underexaggerated ability to shut down the stress response (which causes cortisol levels to remain elevated for longer than they should).

STRESS, CORTISOL, AND METABOLISM

This is probably as good a place as any to introduce the concept that cortisol is not a purely toxic substance—although in most cases too much of it certainly wreaks bodily havoc. In many ways, cortisol can be thought of as functioning like cholesterol or insulin: A small amount of each of these substances is needed for proper functioning. Cholesterol is needed for steroid metabolism. Insulin is necessary for blood-sugar control. And cortisol is needed for the restoration of energy stores following stress. However, if levels of any of these vital compounds exceed a certain small amount for any significant amount of time, you run into problems (blocked arteries in the case of high cholesterol, diabetes in the case of elevated insulin, and obesity and a host of chronic diseases in the case of cortisol).

The whole point here is *balance*—keeping cortisol levels from falling too low or rising too high. In a condition called *Addison's disease*, people are unable to secrete glucocorticoids (such as cortisol) from the adrenal glands. As a result of this inability to mount an effective stress response, people with Addison's disease basically go into a state of shock when faced with a stressful event (they undergo a drop in blood pressure, circulatory collapse, etc.). So just as you do not want cortisol levels to rise too high, neither do you want them to drop too low.

Whenever you're exposed to stress, be it physical stress such as exercise, or emotional stress such as the kind caused by that guy cutting you off in rush-hour traffic, your body begins a complex cascade of events that can alter metabolism in a number of significant ways. Think again about the fight-or-flight mechanism, wherein stimulatory hormones are secreted to prepare the body for rapid action against (fight) or away from (flight) a particular stressor. In a similar manner, upon exposure to everyday stressors the human body also ramps up production of cortisol through a complicated series of events that involves both the hypothalamus and the pituitary glands in the brain (more on that later).

One of cortisol's many functions is that it stimulates the release of glucose, fats, and amino acids for energy production. In the liver, cortisol stimulates the breakdown of glycogen into glucose. In the adipose tissue (where we store body fat), fatty acids are released in response to cortisol stimulation (fat breakdown?—sounds good—but the longer-term effect is fat gain). In the skeletal muscles, cortisol promotes the release of amino acids, which are either used directly by the muscle for energy or sent to the liver for conversion into glucose. The main problem with this last scenario, however, is that if it continues for any prolonged period of time, a significant amount of muscle mass may be lost (bad for long-term weight maintenance).

STRESS AND DISEASE

Scientific research and medical evidence clearly show that a sustained high level of cortisol, coming from chronic unrelenting stress, has a debilitating effect on long-term health. Among these many effects is an increase in appetite and cravings for certain foods. Because one of the primary roles of cortisol is to encourage the body to refuel itself after responding to a stressor, an elevated cortisol level keeps your appetite ramped up—so that you feel hungry almost all the time. In addition, the type of fat that accumulates as a result of this stress-induced appetite will typically locate itself in the abdominal region of the body (probably so it is readily available for the next stress response). The major problem with abdominal fat, aside from the fact that nobody wants a pot belly, is that this type of fat is also highly associated with the development of heart disease, diabetes, and cancer.

Researchers from around the world have slowly been uncovering the relationship between elevated cortisol levels and numerous chronic diseases (listed in the sidebar). Because of the complex relationships between lifestyle, physiology, and psychology, it is not always possible to determine whether elevated cortisol levels are the primary cause of the disease or a mediating factor in the body's response to the disease. For example, a powerful synthetic form of cortisol, called *cortisone*, is used as a drug to reduce swelling, inflammation, and joint pain in rheumatoid arthritis

Elevated cortisol levels resulting from chronic stress have been associated with the following conditions:

- increased appetite and food cravings
- increased body fat
- decreased muscle mass
- decreased bone density
- increased anxiety
- increased depression
- mood swings (anger and irritability)
- reduced libido (sex drive)
- impaired immune response
- memory and learning impairment
- increased symptoms of PMS—premenstrual syndrome (cramps, appetite)
- increased menopausal side effects (hot flashes, night sweats)

(and it performs these actions quite effectively). The catch here is that cortisone use is typically limited to a short period of time, because long-term exposure leads to memory problems, weight gain, depression, and increased infections—making some people feel that they'd be better off with the painful swollen joints instead of the long-term side effects of the drug.

COUNTERACTING THE
EFFECTS OF CHRONIC STRESS

So who has elevated cortisol levels? Lots of people. But to narrow it down, the Stress Self-Test included in the Preface provides a convenient and fairly reliable gauge of a person's exposure to stress and, consequently, of their risk for elevated cortisol levels. Take that test to determine whether you're a Strained Jane, a Stressed Jess, or a Relaxed Jack. Discovering this basic information is a first step in figuring out what you can do to counteract the effects of chronic stress. As mentioned earlier in the chapter, there are numerous approaches for doing so.

For example, many forms of stress management exist, and there are many fine references available on that topic (see the Resources section at the back of the book for a selected listing). This book takes the view that although stress-management techniques have been around for decades, very few of those regimens have made a large impact on the health or well-being of the average person. Why is this true? Are the techniques ineffective? No, many of them work perfectly well—if you can put them into practice. For the vast majority of people, however, wedging another stress-management tool into their already busy life does little more than add further stress. From a purely practical point of view, most people can't be bothered with traditional approaches to stress management. Many of us can't even be bothered to exercise or eat the way we know we should—both of which could go a long way toward reducing the detrimental effects of stress on our bodies.

So what else can we do? Lots! Reading *The Cortisol Connection* is a good start. First we lay the foundation: Chapters 2 through 4 flesh out the relationship between modern lifestyles, stress, cortisol, and a wide range of health problems. Next, the book focuses on presenting ways to counteract stress and the damaging effects of cortisol. It starts in Chapter 5 with an introduction to the SENSE program. SENSE stands for the five key methods for dealing with stress: stress management, exercise, nutrition, supplements, and evaluation.

A prominent focus of this book is on the use of dietary supplements. Specifically, Chapters 6 through 11 outline the supplements that are known to influence stress and cortisol levels. Chapter 6 describes some of the key supplements to *avoid* (because they can *increase* cortisol levels); Chapter 7 covers vitamins and minerals for general stress adaptation; Chapter 8 deals with supplements that offer specific cortisol-control effects; Chapter 9 summarizes adaptogens with wide-ranging "antistress" actions; Chapter 10 focuses on supplements for relaxation and "calming"; and Chapter 11 discusses support supplements that help to control blood sugar, maintain muscle mass, and enhance immune-system function. Each supplement is described in terms of the scientific and medical evidence for its effects on increasing or decreasing cortisol levels. Recommendations for safety, dosage levels, and what to look for if you decide to use the supplement are also provided. These information-rich chapters can be thought of as sort of a handbook of supplements for cortisol control. Some readers will prefer to use this portion of the book as a reference they consult as needed, while others will read it straight through to gain as much knowledge as possible about their different options for cortisol control.

Whichever way you decide to use those chapters, Chapter 12 brings all of the information together in a detailed discussion of the SENSE program. There you will read about three people, Jayne, Marta, and Mario, who used SENSE to literally transform their lives (making "sense" out of them, so to speak).

Besides the three success stories featured in Chapter 12, *The Cortisol Connection* includes several case studies of individuals who have experienced benefits from using diet, exercise, and nutritional supplements to control their cortisol levels. Perhaps you will relate to one or more of these people as experiencing some of the same stressors and life situations as you do—and perhaps some aspects of their approach to cortisol control will help you come up with your own cortisol-control plan.

WHY SUPPLEMENTS?

Why *not* supplements? A strategic regimen of carefully chosen dietary supplements can help control stress, reduce cortisol levels, provide relaxation and more restful sleep, help balance blood sugar, promote weight loss, and boost the immune system. For most of us, from a purely practical perspective, following a balanced cortisol-control regimen that incorporates appropriate dietary supplements is a lot more doable than a complicated stress-management program or a time-consuming exercise regimen. This does not imply that stress management is unimportant or that supplements can provide all of the same benefits delivered by exercise. It simply means that supplements, for the majority of people, represent something that they can realistically incorporate into their already busy daily lives and that can have a powerful beneficial impact on controlling stress and balancing cortisol levels.

Many of the dietary supplements covered in this book have been used for centuries to provide the health benefits described in the preceding paragraph. In some cases the modern scientific evidence for a beneficial health effect of these supplements is quite strong, while in other cases the evidence is weak or nonexistent. The appropriate chapters in this book will guide you through the supplements that appear to hold the most promise in terms of controlling the stress response and counteracting some of the detrimental effects of chronically elevated cortisol.

Summary

After reading this chapter, you are probably more than a little concerned about your future health—and you should be. However, instead of letting concern grow into worry and worry grow into stress, you can do something about your situation.

Maybe you just need to eat better. Or maybe you could benefit from a balanced multivitamin tablet. Perhaps you could use a specific cortisol-controlling supplement—or even an entire program designed to control your stress and cortisol levels. Whatever your individual cortisol-control needs happen to be, the information in this book will help you address them. Your first step toward improved health and lifelong wellness starts on the next page. Good luck!

CHAPTER 2

The Science of Stress

B ecause our modern world rarely requires the evolutionary fight-or-flight response to stress, we deny our bodies their natural physical reaction to stress. Unfortunately, the brain still registers stress in the same way as it always has, but because we no longer react to that stress with vigorous physical activity (fighting or running away), our bodies store the stress response and continue to churn out high levels of stress hormones. Before we know it, we're living the Type C lifestyle, characterized by chronic stress and consistently elevated cortisol levels.

In one of the more ironic twists visited upon us humans as "higher" animals, our brains are so "well developed" that our bodies have learned to respond to *psychological* stress with the same hormonal cascade that happens with exposure to a *physical* stressor. This means that just by our thinking about a stressful event—even if that event is highly unlikely to actually occur—our endocrine system gets all in an uproar. Bad news to be sure—but the upside to this story is that even though psychological variables can trigger the stress response, good evidence exists that we can also harness the mind to counteract some aspects of the stress response, using biofeedback and similar relaxation techniques.

STAGES OF STRESS

When the brain perceives a stressful event, it responds by stimu-lating hormonal (endocrine) glands throughout the body to release hormones, including both adrenaline and cortisol. Adrenaline is responsible for the "up" feeling that causes excite-ment, while cortisol is responsible for modulating the way our bodies use various fuel sources. Cortisol is known as a *glucocorti-coid* because it is secreted by the adrenal cortex (thus *corticoid*) and because it increases levels of blood sugar, or glucose (thus *gluco*corticoid).

The work of the scientist and "father" of stress research, Hans Selye, provides some of the earliest evidence of what we now know as the classic model for adaptation to stress. He observed in rats that given *any* source of external biological stress, an organ-ism would respond with a predictable biological pattern in an attempt to restore its internal homeostasis. In other words, if stress knocks us out of balance, then our bodies will go through a series of steps (the stress response) to help us regain that balance. He termed this struggle to maintain balance the *general adaptation syndrome*, and although modern stress researchers do not agree with every detail of Selye's stress paradigm, his original division of the stress response into three categories is useful for our purposes in understanding what we can do to combat stress.

Selye proposed that the general adaptation syndrome was the body's way of reacting to a stressor (which knocks us out of bal-ance in one way or another) to bring the body's systems back into balance. The first phase of the response, termed the *alarm* phase, is characterized by an immediate activation of the nervous system and adrenal glands; this is the sudden "jolt" that a stressor deliv-ers to the body. Next comes a phase of *resistance*, which is charac-terized by activation of the hypothalamic-pituitary-adrenal (HPA) axis. The HPA axis is the coordinated system of the three primary endocrine tissues (glands) that mediates our response to stress— in other words, the HPA axis is the "machinery" that helps the body "do its thing" when stress occurs.

So far, everything is perfectly normal: Stress happens and the body reacts immediately (alarm phase) to get things moving, and then on a more long-term basis (resistance phase) to restore balance. The problems start to occur when we ask the body to react too often (too much alarm) or with excessive exuberance (too much resistance)—both of which lead us down the path of having elevated cortisol levels. Under these circumstances, when stress is repeated or constant, cortisol levels go up and stay up—causing a third phase of the general adaptation syndrome that is often referred to as *overload*. In this overload stage, bodily systems start to break down and our risk for chronic disease skyrockets. This is when we begin to see problems associated with weight gain, immune-system suppression, depression and anxiety, lack of energy, and inability to concentrate. If the overload phase lasts for a prolonged period of time, we can find ourselves in a serious situation, characterized by gastrointestinal ulceration, widespread tissue dysfunction, and profound metabolic derangement.

ACUTE VERSUS CHRONIC STRESS

This academic discussion of the various stages of the stress response in a bunch of lab rats is all very interesting (really!), but you're probably asking yourself, "What does this all mean for me?" Well, it could mean a great deal—especially when you understand how your own body responds to stress, and whether that stress is encountered acutely or chronically. First, let's take a look at what happens inside the body when stress hits. The body's initial response to a perceived acute stressor is the already mentioned fight-or-flight response that we've lived with since the caveman days. When stress hits, the body's energy reserves (fat, protein, and carbohydrates) are rapidly mobilized (through catabolic breakdown of tissues) to deal with the stressor. Levels of adrenaline and cortisol increase, while DHEA (dehydroepiandrosterone) and testosterone decrease. (The combined effects of high cortisol and low DHEA lead to muscle loss and fat gain—more on that later.)

Common health effects of dealing with acute stressors typically include increased heart rate and blood pressure, increased breathing rate, increased body temperature and sweating, feelings of anxiety and nervousness, headaches, heartburn, and irritability; these are the things you'll feel while the hormones and neurotransmitters rage around in your body. The good news about an acute stressor, however, is that because our energy stores are mobilized to either fight off or get away from the stressor, we can use that energy and heightened alertness to do something good—such as exercise. Unfortunately, if we can't eliminate or escape from the stressor (or use exercise to fool our body into thinking that we're escaping), then the acute stressor quickly becomes a *chronic* stressor.

As the acute stressor becomes more of a chronic stressor, cortisol levels continue to increase and DHEA levels continue to decrease. (There is no rule of thumb for when acute crosses the line into chronic, as it differs widely among people.) As mentioned above, the dual effect of high cortisol and low DHEA leads to muscle loss and fat gain, but it can also have detrimental effects on bone and other tissues (via accelerated breakdown and delayed repair). Typical symptoms associated with chronic stress may include weight gain, fatigue, fluctuations in blood sugar, increased appetite, carbohydrate cravings, muscle weakness, and reduced immune-system function. The loss of muscle tissue leads to a fall in basal metabolic rate (the number of calories the body burns at rest) and marks the turning point between "early" and "late" chronic stress, sometimes called *Stage 2* and *Stage 3* stress by researchers. The early stages of chronic stress can be considered more of a *hypercatabolic* situation, characterized by accelerated tissue destruction, whereas the later stages put a person into more of a *hypoanabolic* state, where the ability to rebuild vital tissues is impaired. At this later stage, much of the damage has already been done—so muscle and bone tissues are weaker, sex drive is reduced (because of low DHEA, growth hormone, and sex steroids), and the person is entering a vicious cycle of increased appetite, reduced caloric expenditure, and accelerated fat accumulation.

The bottom line here is that the body can deal with acute stress, and it can do so with great effectiveness as long as the acute stress is dealt with *before* it progresses into the chronic stages. How? By exercising. As the Nike ads used to say about exercise, "Just do it!"—because doing so will be your best hedge against acute stress slipping into the realm of chronic stress (more on exercise appears in Chapters 5 and 12).

But now let's get real. If we all had the time, resources, and inclination to "just do it" on a regular basis, there would be a lot fewer people reading this book (or at least a few more reading it while on their treadmills). The reality is, however, that most of us (this author included) cannot simply drop what we are doing and run off to "do it" (exercise, that is) at a moment's notice. So we miss a few (or more than a few) exercise sessions, our acute stressors "build up" in a sense, and we slowly slip into the initial stages of chronic stress.

INDIVIDUAL RESPONSES TO STRESS

Okay, so now you know that stress exerts a disruptive influence on the body and that one of these effects is an increase in the release of cortisol. It is important to note, however, that a huge difference exists between people in their individual ability to tolerate a given amount of stress. Some people can simply "take" a greater load of stress before they begin to break down. That said, even some of the toughest and most "stress-resistant" individuals on the planet, such as Marine Corps recruits, will still succumb to the adverse effects of stress. In one study, military recruits were subjected to five days of extreme exercise, starvation, and sleep deprivation. Not surprisingly, due to the stressful nature of this training, cortisol levels went up and performance deteriorated. The researchers also found that even after five days of rest and refueling, cortisol levels still had not returned to normal—demonstrating the fact that no matter how tough and stress-resistant you think you may be, even *you* have a breaking point.

In another study, this one of Swedish factory workers, differences in the stress response were compared between men and women. The researchers showed that although both male and female workers endured similar levels of stress while at work, stress levels in men fell off quickly when they left work. In contrast, stress levels among the female workers tended to either remain the same or even increase when they left work—suggesting that the women continued to be exposed to high levels of stress hormones while they looked after their family and household responsibilities (so much for gender equality).

In addition to the stress faced by Marine recruiters and Swedish workers, stress researchers frequently study competitive athletes. For obvious reasons, athletes are extremely interested in balancing the "dose" of stress they deliver to their bodies with the amount of recovery necessary for optimal performance. Counteracting the muscle-wasting and fat-gaining effects of prolonged cortisol exposure becomes a large part of maximizing performance gains while minimizing the risk for injury. For many athletes, the delicate balance of training and recovery poses a significant dilemma: To go fast, you have to train hard, but training too hard without adequate recovery will just make you slow, because you'll be tired or get hurt. Athletes who excel, however, are those who are most adept at balancing the three primary components of their program: training, diet, and recovery. A phenomenon known as *overtraining* syndrome has been linked to chronic cortisol exposure—exactly the same situation that we all face in our battle with daily stressors. Although chronic overtraining is easy to recognize by its common symptoms of constant fatigue, mood fluctuations, and reduced mental and physical performance (sound familiar?), it may be difficult to detect in its earlier stages—just like the early stages of stress. Therefore, competitive athletes, just like each of us, need to become adept at balancing *exposure* to stress with *recovery* from stress in order to approach the optimal physical and mental performance we're all looking for.

──────────────── Summary ────────────────

That's the general overview of the stress response. Acute stress followed by adequate adaptation leads to optimal long-term health. On the other hand, chronic stress followed by insufficient adaptation leads to metabolic disturbances, tissue breakdown, and chronic disease.

We all know that stress is "bad" for us—even our grandmothers knew this and their grandmothers before them. But why? The next chapter outlines some of the latest scientific theories and medical evidence suggesting that a large part of the detrimental effects of chronic stress on health may be due to the primary stress hormone: cortisol.

CHAPTER 3

All About Cortisol, the Master Stress Hormone

If you've been paying attention throughout the first two chapters, then you already know the basic relationship between stress and cortisol. For those who missed it, stress makes cortisol levels go up. You also understand that cortisol can be both a "good thing" and a "bad thing"—depending on how much cortisol is present in the body and how long it hangs around. In very general terms, cortisol turns "bad" when you either have too much of it or get exposed to it on a regular basis. What follows in this chapter is a closer look at the dynamics of cortisol metabolism. This chapter will serve as a primer to the next one, which outlines some of the emerging research into the relationship between stress, cortisol, and many of the chronic diseases of our modern society.

THE ENDOCRINE SYSTEM

The vast network of hormones and glands in the body is known as the *endocrine system*. This system is made up of specialized tissues (glands) that play an integral part in our overall response to stress. Through our senses of sight, sound, smell, and even our thoughts, the brain collects information and uses both the nervous system and the endocrine system to respond to what it "observes" in the environment. When we encounter a stressor, whether through our physical or our psychological senses, the endocrine system jumps into action to set things right. Through the coordinated actions of two glands in the brain (the hypothalamus and the pituitary), along with another set of glands that sit just above the kidneys (the adrenal glands), stress causes a cascade of hormonal signals to be set in motion. These hormonal signals involve epinephrine (adrenaline), norepinephrine, cortisol, and numerous intermediary hormones that interact to help regulate important aspects of physiology such as cardiovascular function, energy metabolism, immune-system activity, and brain chemistry.

THE ADRENAL GLANDS

The two adrenal glands are located just above the kidneys (Figure 3.1). Each adrenal gland is made up of two parts—the inner medulla, which produces adrenaline, and the outer cortex, which produces cortisol and aldosterone (another steroid hormone that is important in salt/water balance and blood pressure). Cortisol and other glucocorticoids are secreted in response to stimulation of the adrenal glands by adrenocorticotropic hormone (ACTH, also known as *corticotropin*) from the pituitary gland. Secretion of ACTH is under the control of another hormone from the hypothalamus called *corticotropin-releasing hormone* (CRH).

It is easy to see how closely the central nervous system is linked with the endocrine (hormone) system. The brain perceives stress; it responds by secreting CRH from the hypothalamus in the brain; CRH stimulates the pituitary gland (also in the brain) to secrete ACTH; and ACTH travels to the adrenal glands (on top of the kidneys) to stimulate cortisol production.

Cortisol levels typically fluctuate in a fairly rhythmic fashion throughout the day, with the highest levels in the morning and

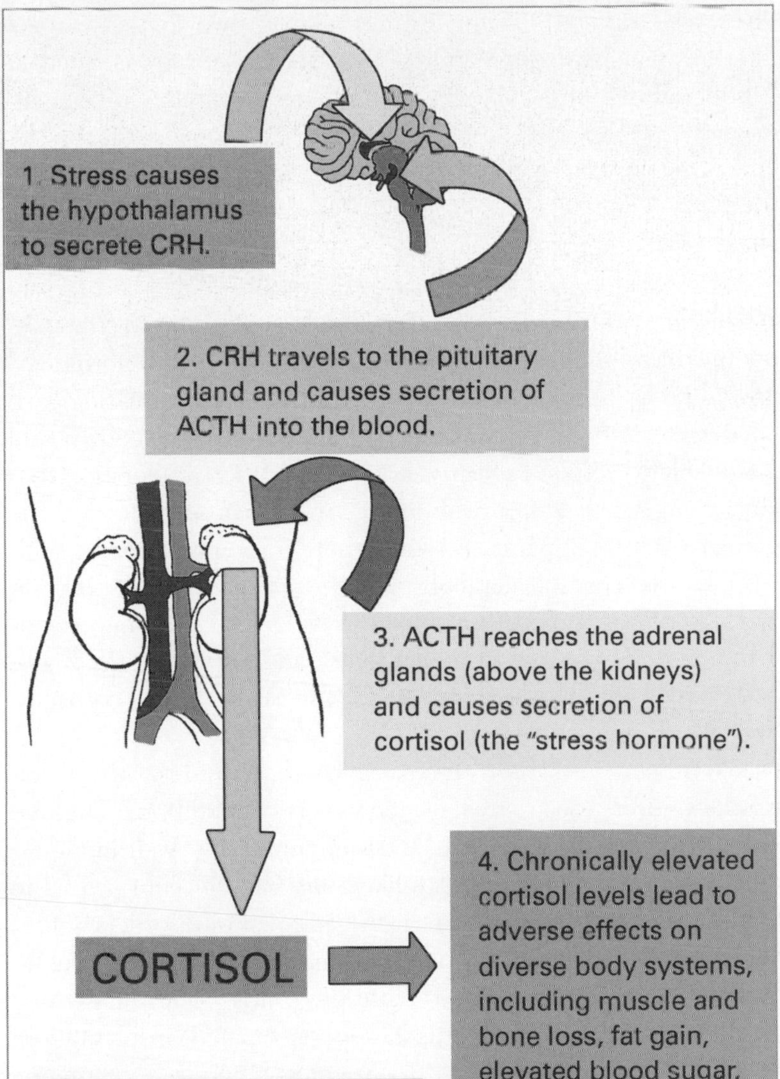

1. Stress causes the hypothalamus to secrete CRH.

2. CRH travels to the pituitary gland and causes secretion of ACTH into the blood.

3. ACTH reaches the adrenal glands (above the kidneys) and causes secretion of cortisol (the "stress hormone").

CORTISOL

4. Chronically elevated cortisol levels lead to adverse effects on diverse body systems, including muscle and bone loss, fat gain, elevated blood sugar, high blood pressure, suppressed immuno-system function, and changes in memory and mood.

Figure 3.1: Hormonal cascade caused by stress

CRH = corticotropin-releasing hormone; ACTH = adrenocor-ticotropic hormone (also known as corticotropin)

the lowest at night. It is important to note, however, that cortisol
rhythms can be disrupted by a wide variety of factors, such as
emotional and physical stress, inadequate sleep, and various illnesses.

WHAT IS CORTISOL?

Cortisol, also known as *cortisone* and *hydrocortisone*, is a steroid
hormone produced in the adrenal glands in response to stress. As
such, cortisol is often referred to as the primary "stress hormone."
In the body, cortisol is needed to maintain normal physiological
processes during times of stress; without cortisol, the body would
be unable to respond effectively to stress. Without cortisol, that
lion charging at us from the bushes would cause us to do little
more than wet our pants and stand there staring (not good). With
an effective cortisol metabolism, however, we're primed to run
away or do battle, because cortisol secretion releases amino acids
(from muscle), glucose (from the liver), and fatty acids (from adipose tissue) into the bloodstream for use as energy. So cortisol is
"good"—right? Yes. And no.

Synthetic forms of cortisol, such as prednisone and dexa-
methasone, are used to treat a wide variety of conditions. They are
usually prescribed for their anti-inflammatory and immune-
suppressing properties. Cortisol-like drugs can be quite helpful in
relieving excessive inflammation in certain skin disorders (Pfizer
makes an anti-itch skin cream called CortiZone), as well as in
inflammatory diseases such as arthritis, colitis, or asthma (those
inhalers contain corticosteroids). During organ transplantation,
cortisol-like drugs are used to suppress the body's immune
response and help reduce the chance of the body's rejecting the
newly transplanted organ. Cortisol-like drugs are also used as
replacement therapy for people who have lost function of their
adrenal glands (Addison's disease). So, again, cortisol is a "good
thing"—right? Yes, but only at certain levels and for a certain
period of time.

WHAT DOES CORTISOL DO?

Cortisol has diverse and highly important effects on regulating aspects of all parts of the body's metabolism of glucose, protein, and fatty acids. The functions of cortisol are also particularly important in controlling mood and well-being, immune cells and inflammation, blood vessels and blood pressure, and the maintenance of connective tissues such as bones, muscles, and skin. Under conditions of stress, cortisol normally maintains blood pressure and limits excessive inflammation. Unfortunately, many people's adrenal stress response overreacts by secreting too much cortisol—with devastating consequences.

Cortisol and related corticoids are also known as *glucocorticoids*, a term that, as was pointed out in the preceding chapter, is derived from early scientific observations that these hormones are intimately involved in glucose metabolism. Cortisol is known to stimulate several metabolic processes that collectively serve to increase concentrations of glucose in blood.

These effects include stimulation of gluconeogenesis (conversion of amino acids into glucose), mobilization of amino acids from muscle tissues (to serve as the raw material in gluconeogenesis), inhibition of glucose uptake in muscle and adipose (fat) tissue (which further increases blood-sugar levels), and stimulation of fat breakdown in adipose tissue. Unfortunately, the fatty acids released by lipolysis (fat breakdown) have a detrimental effect on health by reducing cellular sensitivity to insulin, a condition that can be a precursor to diabetes. Cortisol also has potent anti-inflammatory and immunosuppressive properties—both of which are important in regulating normal responses of the immune system.

THE GOOD, THE BAD, AND THE UGLY OF CORTISOL METABOLISM

The preceding few paragraphs certainly place cortisol in a positive light by focusing on the "good" aspects of cortisol metabolism—and they outline exactly what we would expect from a "normal" pattern of cortisol metabolism (that is, in a perfect world). In that perfect world, cortisol metabolism would look something like this: A stressor is encountered, the endocrine system is activated, the stressor is dealt with, and the stress response is ended. All in all a very simple reaction. However, when the endocrine system becomes either *over*activated or is activated *chronically* (on a regular or repeated basis), the result can be an overall dysregulation of the endocrine system that can lead to a gradual and progressive deterioration of general health and a worsening of existing conditions.

So why even have a stress response if it causes so many problems? Good question. Back in our "caveman" days, this stress response was a vital survival technique—and *not* having such a response would have meant that we were easy prey for saber-toothed tigers and other predators. To repeat how all this works (because this is such an important part of understanding the health problems that arise from chronic stress), the stress response involves a brief increase in energy levels, hormone levels, and ability for forceful muscle contraction—otherwise known as the *fight-or-flight* mechanism. The phrase fight or flight means just what it says: It prepares the body to deal with the stressor by either attacking it or running away from it. Unfortunately, even in these modern times, when we're faced with a "benign" stressor, such as a project deadline or a traffic jam (these may be irritating, but they're not going to swallow you like the aforementioned tiger), our bodies undergo the very same metabolic stress changes—which can lead us down the path to increased disease risks.

Under normal circumstances, the body does a pretty good job of controlling cortisol secretion and regulating the amount of cortisol in the bloodstream—but not always (more on that later). Normal cortisol metabolism follows a circadian rhythm (Figure 3.2)—meaning that levels tend to follow a twenty-four-hour cycle—with the highest cortisol levels typically observed in the early morning (about 6:00 to 8:00 A.M.) and the lowest levels in the wee hours of the morning (about midnight to 2:00 A.M.). Cortisol levels usually show a rapid drop between 8:00 A.M. and

11:00 A.M., and a continued gradual decline throughout the day. From those lowest levels around 2:00 A.M., cortisol again begins to rise to help us wake up and prepare for another stressful day.

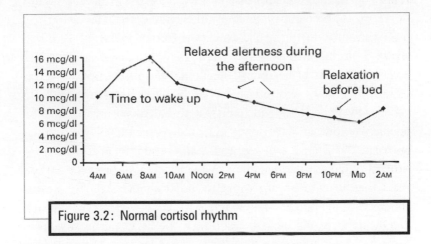

16 mcg/dl
14 mcg/dl
12 mcg/dl
10 mcg/dl
8 mcg/dl
6 mcg/dl
4 mcg/dl
2 mcg/dl
0

4AM 6AM 8AM 10AM NOON 2PM 4PM 6PM 8PM 10PM MID 2AM

Time to wake up

Relaxed alertness during the afternoon

Relaxation before bed

Figure 3.2: Normal cortisol rhythm

It is interesting to note that people who work the graveyard shift for prolonged periods of time (more than a year) undergo alterations in their "cortisol clocks." Their cortisol levels are lowest during the day (when they get their deepest sleep) and start to rise again in late afternoon to early evening when they must get up and get ready for their night work. This is exactly opposite from the pattern we see in people with "normal" work schedules. However, it is important to note that most shift workers (those who pick up an occasional late shift now and again) show no such adaptation in cortisol metabolism. For these people, the additional late shift merely disrupts sleep patterns and keeps cortisol elevated when it should be falling.

The "normal" range for blood cortisol levels is fairly wide, 6–23 mcg/dl (micrograms per deciliter), but these levels can vary tremendously in response to stress, illness, and even following meals (each of which increases cortisol levels). Urinary levels of cortisol have an even wider range of "normal" values (10–100 mcg/24 hours), but this measurement at least avoids some of the large variations in cortisol levels seen throughout the day. Cortisol levels can also be elevated by estrogen hormone therapy, exercise, pregnancy, depression, anxiety, and even by the intake of mild stimulants such as ephedra (used for weight loss) or caffeine (as little as two to three cups of coffee will elevate cortisol levels).

Now, for some of the *bad* aspects of cortisol metabolism. If the above information makes you think that your "normal" cortisol levels are at risk for becoming elevated, then you're not alone. In fact, with today's Western lifestyles being defined by our fast-paced, low-sleep, fast-food habits, it would be surprising to find people who did *not* experience elevated cortisol levels on a regular basis. "So what," you say? You're not afraid of no stinkin' cortisol? Well, you should be. Here's why, to reemphasize yet another point that bears repeating from the earlier chapters: There is very good scientific and medical evidence to show that chronically elevated cortisol levels are associated with obesity, hypertension, diabetes, fatigue, depression, moodiness, irregular menstrual periods, decreased sex drive, and Alzheimer's disease.

Whenever our bodies are exposed to a stressor, cortisol springs into action to increase levels of fat and sugar in the bloodstream—which can be used by the brain and muscles to deal with the stressor. Normally, cortisol levels are quickly depleted following the stress response. Unfortunately, the way our bodies were designed to deal with stress (fight or flight) is not the way we deal with stress in our modern world, where we simply try to ignore the stress hormones pulsing through our bodies. This scenario means that our bodies are unable to deplete their stores of stress hormones—which induces even more stress and stimulates an even more pronounced secretion of cortisol.

Because our bodies were meant to deal only with immediate short-term exposure to stress hormones, this chronic long-term exposure to cortisol can quickly lead to breakdowns in the body's metabolic control systems. Most of the problems associated with elevated cortisol levels have their origins in a disrupted metabolism, causing elevations in blood sugar, cholesterol, blood pressure, and body-fat levels. This cluster of related metabolic disturbances is termed the *metabolic syndrome*, or sometimes *syndrome X*. Many people with syndrome X are easily recognizable because of their accumulation of abdominal body fat (they look apple-shaped) and their high waist-to-hip ratio (WHR). Research has clearly shown that the higher a person's WHR (the bigger one's waist circumference compared to his or her hip circumference), the higher his or her risk for developing syndrome X. An optimal WHR is usually considered anything under 0.8 (meaning a smaller waist than hip circumference), while anything over 0.85 puts a person at risk for syndrome X (more on syndrome X in the next chapter).

Recall from Chapter 1 (in the section titled "Stress and Disease") how one of the most notable effects of chronically elevated cortisol levels is an increase in appetite and cravings for certain foods. These cravings tend to be for calorie-dense sweets and salty snacks—and this illustrates in one more way the fact that human beings were simply not meant to carry around constant disturbances in our stress response (chronic stress); we were built to respond to stress quickly and then to have those stress hormones dissipate immediately. When our bodies are exposed to wave after wave of the stress that comes from modern lifestyles, our bodies gradually begin to break down. Animals simply don't normally harbor chronic stress the way humans do.

THE CATABOLIC EFFECTS OF CHRONICALLY ELEVATED CORTISOL

Too much cortisol for too long a period of time leads from the merely "bad" to the downright "ugly" aspects of cortisol overexposure. This ugly phase is characterized by widespread tissue destruction and system breakdown (also referred to as *catabolism*), such as muscle loss, bone loss, immune-system suppression, and brain shrinkage.

For example, very brief exposure to cortisol, such as during periods of acute fight-or-flight stress, causes an initial stimulation of immune-system activity and mental ability (good things if you are trying to evade a predator). Even this initial stimulatory effect of cortisol can *over*activate the immune system in some people, leading to allergies, asthma, and various autoimmune diseases such as rheumatoid arthritis, lupus, and fibromyalgia (all of which are known to be triggered by stressful events). On the other hand, however, a more chronic, longer-term exposure to cortisol has the opposite effect, causing immune cells to die and *in*activating our immune-system protection.

These phenomena are explained in more detail in the next chapter, where we see the wide-ranging health effects of cortisol overexposure.

Summary

So there you have it. The "good" aspects of cortisol, such as its anti-inflammatory benefits, are great to have around—but only for a short period of time in very specific situations. But we all have stress. And those of us who endure repeated stress, or hectic lifestyles, or are dieting, or sleep less than eight hours per night are likely to have chronic stress—and chronically elevated cortisol levels. This is when the "bad" aspects of cortisol begin to appear, as metabolic changes that include elevated blood sugar, increased appetite, accelerated weight gain, reduced sex drive, and severe fatigue. Left untreated, these conditions can lead to truly "ugly" problems such as muscle and bone loss, immune-system breakdown, and brain shrinkage.

Given the above information, it is vitally important for each of us to approach control of our cortisol levels as a primary focus for achieving long-term health and well-being. The next chapter deals with the relationship between stress, cortisol, and disease and will help set the stage for you to make meaningful steps toward improving how you feel, how you look, and your risk for certain diseases.

CHAPTER 4

The Relationship Between Stress, Cortisol, and Disease

So now you know a bit about how chronic stress leads to elevated cortisol levels in the body. This chapter details the next piece of the puzzle: the relationship between those elevated cortisol levels and the risk for a wide range of chronic diseases. It should come as no big surprise to anybody reading this book that the effects of stress on a person's long-term health can be far-reaching. The medical literature tells us quite clearly that many of the conditions associated with a "modern" lifestyle—conditions such as obesity, diabetes, hypertension, insomnia, headaches, ulcers, depression, anxiety, poor memory, and a lower resistance to infections—are all related to high stress levels. Also noteworthy is the consistent finding that people dramatically increase their use of the medical system during times of heightened stress (such as job insecurity) and that there is a tight association between elevated cortisol levels and higher health-care costs. In such cases, episodes of illness, doctor visits, and trips to hospital outpatient departments have been shown to double (at least) when compared to lower-stress periods of time. We see the same pattern emerge during final-exam week on college campuses, when walk-in health clinics are filled with sick students during their most stressed-out time of the year. Other evidence clearly demonstrates that workers reporting the highest level of perceived stress due to job dissatisfaction, family problems, and personal conflict are the most likely to experience somatic symptoms such as colds, flu, allergies, asthma, and headaches.

METABOLIC CONSEQUENCES
OF ELEVATED CORTISOL LEVELS

Okay, so cortisol is toxic—right? Not so fast. As we know from the previous chapters, cortisol is a vital hormone; without it, the body would be ill prepared to deal with the stresses of daily life. On the other hand, excess cortisol secretion and chronically elevated cortisol levels can lead to a host of related metabolic disturbances and an increased risk for developing a variety of chronic conditions. We touched on many of these effects in the preceding chapters, and they are summarized here in Table 4.1.

Stress-related diseases occur because of an excessive activation of the stress response in the brain and in the endocrine (hormone) system to common, everyday sources of physical and psychological stress. The various stressors to which we are all subjected each day can disrupt the body's stable balance of temperature, blood pressure, and other functions. Unfortunately, as mentioned before, because the human brain is so well developed, it can also respond to *imagined* stress with the very same stress response that is supposed to be reserved for life-or-death (fight-or-flight) situations. Accordingly, injury, hunger, heat, cold, or worry can trigger the stress response just as would happen if you were running for your life or fighting off an attacker.

In 1999, a team of Swedish researchers showed that exposure to high levels of stress caused a rapid increase in cortisol secretion, followed by reduced sex-hormone levels and depressed libido (sex drive). That same year, a report from the New York Academy of Sciences suggested that elevated cortisol

Table 4.1: Metabolic and Long-Term Health Effects of Elevated Cortisol Levels

Metabolic Effect (Cortisol-Induced)	Chronic Health Condition
Increased appetite, accelerated muscle catabolism (breakdown), suppressed fat oxidation, enhanced fat storage	Obesity
Elevated cholesterol and triglyceride levels	Heart disease
Elevated blood pressure	Heart disease
Alterations in brain neurochemistry (involving dopamine and serotonin)	Depression/anxiety
Physical atrophy (shrinkage) of brain cells	Alzheimer's disease
Insulin resistance and elevated blood-sugar levels	Diabetes
Accelerated bone resorption (breakdown)	Osteoporosis
Reduced levels of testosterone and estrogen	Suppressed libido (reduced sex drive)
Suppression of immune-cell number and activity	Frequent colds/flu/ infection
Reduced synthesis of brain neurotransmitters	Memory/concentration problems

levels, caused by exposure to perceived stress, was associated with development of the metabolic syndrome (a.k.a. syndrome X) described in the preceding chapter (characterized by insulin resistance, diabetes, abdominal obesity, elevated cholesterol, and hypertension). Research published in 2000 by scientists at Yale University supports the idea that emotional stress contributes to weight gain in both overweight and lean women. The researchers noted that the connection between stress and obesity is most likely due to an excessive secretion of cortisol and the adverse metabolic effects of the hormone in people with chronically elevated levels.

Elevated cortisol levels are also associated with reduced levels of testosterone and IGF-1 in men exposed to high stress; both are considered to be anabolic or muscle-building hormones, so these men also tend to have reduced muscle mass and higher body-fat levels. These same men also tend to have a higher body mass index (BMI), a higher waist-to-hip ratio (WHR), and abdominal obesity (an apple shape). Researchers at the Neurological Institute at the University of California at San Francisco (UCSF) have linked excess cortisol levels to depression, anxiety, and Alzheimer's disease, as well as to direct changes in brain structure (atrophy) leading to cognitive defects (meaning that cortisol can shrink and kill brain cells).

So, as emphasized throughout this book, cortisol is not all bad—but too much of it for too long is a recipe for disaster. The sections that follow will outline in greater detail the metabolic relationship between elevated cortisol and specific conditions. Be warned: The news is not good for those of us who experience stress on a regular basis; the next section may even leave you feeling as if your high stress levels are killing you (and they are!). There is good news, however, and it starts in Chapter 5, where we'll begin to learn about the various steps that can help us get a handle on our stress response and help us modulate cortisol levels within a more healthful range.

HOW STRESS MAKES US FAT:
CORTISOL, DIABETES, AND OBESITY

As a young lawyer early in his career, *Paul* was expected (and quite willing) to work long hours under tight project deadlines, a situation that obviously led to a heightened sense of stress. For a number of years, Paul appeared to be more than able to cope with—and indeed, even to thrive under—his monumental stress load. Unfortunately, as his career advanced, he added not only many new clients (more work), but also a wife and two kids (more commitments), and a vacation home with a sizable mortgage (more financial pressure).

Having been a college athlete, Paul knew the difference between "good" and "bad" nutrition and exercise habits, but no matter what he did with his diet or workout program, he experienced a slow but gradual creeping up of his body weight— and a significant amount of trouble getting rid of that excess weight. He also noticed that on his most stressful days, he found himself craving foods he would ordinarily stay away from (Big Macs and candy bars). To see how Paul successfully conquered his stress-related weight gain, see Chapter 11.

A primary focal point of this book is the close (and increasingly understood) relationship between stress, cortisol, and being overweight or obese. A key intermediary in the relationship is another hormone called *insulin*. Most people associate insulin problems with diabetes because of its primary role in regulating blood-sugar levels (although insulin has many additional functions in the body). Not only does insulin regulate blood-sugar levels within an extremely narrow range; it is also responsible for getting fat stored in our fat cells (adipose tissue), getting sugar stored in our liver and muscle cells (as glycogen), and getting amino acids directed toward protein synthesis (muscle building). Due to these varied actions, insulin is sometimes thought of as a "storage" hormone because it helps the body put all these great sources of energy away in their respective places for use later. That's great, but it is exactly the opposite effect of what the body experiences during the stress response—when the heart and muscles need lots of energy and need it fast.

One of the first signals the body must send out (via cortisol) during periods of stress is one that screams, "No more energy storage!"—and that means shutting off the responsiveness of cells to the storage effects of insulin. When cells stop responding to insulin, they are able to switch from a storage (anabolic/building) mode to a secretion (catabolic/breakdown) mode—so fat cells dump more fat into the system, liver cells crank out more glucose, and muscle cells allow their protein to be broken down to supply amino acids (for conversion into even more sugar by the liver). This is all fine—assuming it occurs infrequently and for only a short period of time. Telling the body's cells to ignore insulin on a regular basis, as happens with chronic stress, can lead to a condition known as *insulin resistance* and predispose a person to the development of full-blown diabetes.

Stress makes a person fat primarily because of an excessive secretion of the key stress hormone, cortisol, along with a reduced secretion of key anabolic hormones, such as DHEA and Growth Hormone. This combination of high cortisol and low DHEA causes the body to store fat, lose muscle, slow metabolic rate, and increase appetite—all of which have the ultimate effect of making a person fatter. Overall, stress makes you burn fewer calories and consume more food (especially carbohydrates)—which increases your stress levels even more! Even the *thought* of food and the *concern* about eating can increase stress—and therefore cortisol—levels in people who have restrained their eating habits and are either dieting or are concerned about their weight.

Scientific studies have shown that chronic stress clearly leads to overeating—which then leads to fat accumulation (frequently in the abdominal area). When we look at the relationship between stress and appetite, the picture can get a bit confusing—but it clears up when we look at the timing of the stress response. In the very early stages of stress, one hormone is secreted that *suppresses* appetite, while later in the stress response, another hormone is secreted to *increase* appetite. You'll remember from earlier chapters that in response to stress, the hypothalamus in the brain gets the stress engines going by secreting CRH (corticotropin-releasing hormone). CRH kills the appetite. Now, before you get all excited and run off to order a month's supply of CRH over the Internet, you should also realize that although having more CRH around would certainly cut your appetite, it would also make you feel like you were having an anxiety or panic attack (not good).

Okay, so CRH *kills* appetite for the first few seconds of the stress response, but hot on its heels comes a dramatic rise in cortisol—which *stimulates* appetite (often by a lot) in the minutes to hours following the stressful event. CRH levels drop back to normal in seconds, while cortisol levels may take many hours to normalize—meaning that your appetite stays ramped up for a very long time (which drives you crazy until you finally succumb and eat something). Thought of in evolutionary terms, cortisol is actually quite a useful little hormone to have around; without it, our appetite would stay suppressed following a stressful event (such as running from the lion) and we'd never have the drive to refuel our depleted body. The obvious downside, of course, is that we're rarely expending huge amounts of energy when dealing with our modern stressors (sitting in a traffic jam doesn't burn very many calories), so the stimulated appetite makes us eat when we're not really hungry—and we get fat.

Researchers have noticed that this pattern of accumulating abdominal fat during periods of stress is quite similar to a disease known as *Cushing's syndrome*, which is characterized by extremely high cortisol levels. In people afflicted with Cushing's syndrome, a prolonged exposure to excessive amounts of cortisol leads to massive accumulations of abdominal fat accompanied by severe loss of muscle tissue in the extremities (arms and legs). Many scientists now understand that the excessive cortisol production and tissue breakdown of Cushing's syndrome is similar in many ways to chronic cortisol exposure caused by repeated periods of stress (which can also lead to losses of vital bone and muscle tissue).

During periods of chronic stress, levels of both cortisol and insulin rise and together send a potent signal to fat cells to store as much fat as possible. They also signal fat cells to hold on to their fat stores—so stress can actually reduce the ability of the body to release fat from its fat stores to use for energy. In terms of weight gain and obesity, the link between cortisol and deranged metabolism is seen in many ways. These are listed in the sidebar below.

Metabolic Effects of Elevated Cortisol (Related to Weight Gain)

Loss of Muscle Mass

- breakdown of muscles, tendons, and ligaments (to provide amino acids for conversion into glucose)
- decreased synthesis of protein (to conserve amino acids for conversion into glucose)
- reduced levels of DHEA, growth hormone, IGF-1, and thyroid-stimulating hormone (TSH)
- drop in basal metabolic rate (i.e., a reduced number of calories is burned throughout the day and night)

Increase in Blood-Sugar Levels

- reduced transport of glucose into cells
- decreased insulin sensitivity
- increase in appetite and carbohydrate cravings

Increase in Body Fat

- increase in the overall amount of body fat (due to increased appetite, overeating, and reduced metabolic rate)
- a redistribution and accumulation of body fat to the abdominal region

From a vanity standpoint, nobody wants to carry around more body fat than they need to. From a health and longevity standpoint, elevated cortisol levels also tend to promote a particular type of fat accumulation (in the abdominal area) that is tightly associated with heart disease, diabetes, hypertension, and high cholesterol. Researchers are not completely sure why this "stress fat" accumulates specifically around the midsection. Its location here may have something to do with its being available for rapid access when the body needs additional fuel (because fat stored in the abdominal region can be delivered to the bloodstream and tissues faster then fat stored in peripheral regions such as the thighs and buttocks). But even though the *reason* for abdominal fat accumulation is still unclear, its *consequences* are well known. This combination of conditions, known as metabolic syndrome or syndrome X (as you may recall from the preceding chapter), has been identified by many experts as the most important health danger that we'll face as a worldwide population in the early twenty-first century. It is covered in more detail in the next section.

Most of us have grown fatter as we've grown older. It is interesting to note that several recent studies have demonstrated quite clearly that cortisol secretion increases with aging, elevated cortisol levels reduce our sensitivity to insulin, and reduced insulin sensitivity is clearly linked to obesity, diabetes, and metabolic syndrome X. In some studies, overweight and obese subjects have been found to have cortisol levels in the normal range prior to meals, but within twenty to forty minutes of eating, with cortisol levels that have surged. This effect of excessive cortisol secretion is also present for lean individuals, but overweight and obese people tend to exhibit the phenomenon to a much greater degree— leading several stress researchers to hypothesize that increased cortisol production may be one of the primary causative factors in weight gain.

There is certainly no shortage of observational studies showing the close relationship between hypercortisolemia (high blood levels of cortisol), hyperinsulinemia (high insulin levels), and reduced growth hormone. It is also interesting (and confusing) to note that some studies find no differences in the *absolute* cortisol levels between obese and lean subjects or between stressed and unstressed volunteers. What these studies *do* show, however, is an alteration in the normal secretory pattern of cortisol. This fluctuating pattern, when normal, should show the highest levels of cortisol in the morning, with a slow and gradual drop toward the lowest levels around 2:00 A.M. (refer back to Figure 3.2 on page 27).

Stressed-out subjects with an altered pattern of cortisol secretion are characterized by a low morning cortisol concentration, the absence of a circadian rhythm, and a huge meal-related surge in cortisol levels (see Figure 4.1)—all of which are consistently associated with obesity and related measurements. People with disrupted cortisol-secretion patterns have higher body fat (particularly in the abdomen), lower muscle mass (particularly in the arms and legs), and reduced basal metabolic rate (BMR, the number of calories burned at rest). On the other hand, the more "normal" pattern of cortisol metabolism (high in the morning, with a normal circadian rhythm) is associated with more favorable measures of body composition (more lean and less fat) as well as a healthier cardiovascular profile (lower blood pressure, reduced cholesterol and blood sugar, and better insulin sensitivity).

All in all, the above scenario makes for a very discouraging scenario: Stress makes us fat. Even worse, however, may be the findings from researchers that have determined that the stress of *dieting* can make us fat. Why is this especially bad news? Primarily because at any given moment in our Western society, as much as 50 to 60 percent of the population is actively dieting—and many millions more are at least concerned about what they eat. This makes dieting one of the most common stress triggers in our modern society (for both men and women)—but why are so many people dieting? Aside from the obvious fact that few of us eat right or exercise enough, we also have to contend with the mass-media messages equating thinness with beauty, success, and intelligence (and the implication that we can't achieve those things unless we

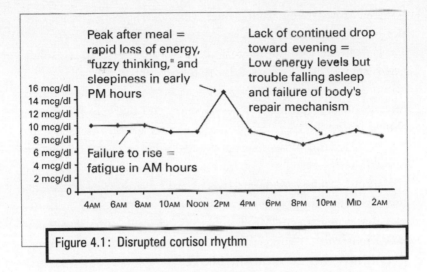

Figure 4.1: Disrupted cortisol rhythm

are thin). Unfortunately, we also have to contend with the very real physiological changes that are occurring within each of us. As we age, our metabolic rate drops and most of us begin to pack on the pounds. Adding fat in the abdominal area (in response to stress) changes the body shape from that of an hourglass to more of a shot glass—and repeated diets only compound the problem.

Most of us will experience a drop in metabolism of about 0.5 percent per year after the age of twenty (largely due to a loss of about five to ten pounds of muscle tissue every decade). Now, that may not seem like a large drop, but when you look at it over ten or twenty years, it means that we're burning 5 percent fewer calories at age thirty and 10 percent fewer calories at age forty—and so it goes, with about 5 percent fewer calories burned for every ten years of age. Just imagine: By the time we turn fifty, we're burning 15 percent fewer calories than we did when we were twenty (Table 4.2). If you consume two thousand calories per day at age twenty (which is about average), this means you will need only seventeen hundred calories (three hundred fewer calories) at age fifty to maintain your body weight. It also means that if you don't make some serious changes in your diet and exercise patterns, or at least get your cortisol levels under control, then your fifty-year-old body will be carrying around over thirty extra pounds of fat than when you were twenty!

Remember that during periods of chronic stress, such as dieting, rising cortisol levels send a potent signal to fat cells, telling them to store as much fat as possible. Cortisol also signals fat cells to hold on to their fat stores—so stress can actually reduce the ability of the body to release fat from its fat stores to use for energy. Does this mean that people with higher levels of stress are less able to lose weight? Yes, for a variety of reasons.

In one study, volunteers took part in a fifteen-week weight-loss program. They were put on a diet of seven hundred calories per day. As expected, the subjects experienced a significant increase in overall hunger, desire to eat, and total food consumption (when they were finally allowed to eat as much as they wanted). The most consistent predictor of these changes in desire to eat, fullness, and food intake was the change (increase) in cortisol levels. The researchers hypothesized that the low-calorie diet induced a form of stress that increased cortisol levels and caused the people in the study to eat more—but it also may have simply been that the dieters were hungry because the researchers were starving them (after all, seven hundred calories per day is not a lot of food). So, to test the theory that the increase in hunger was

Table 4.2: Change in Metabolic Rate and Weight Gain with Age

Age (Years)	Calorie Needs (Daily)	Drop in Daily Metabolic Rate (from Age 20)	Pounds of Extra Fat (from Age 20)*
20	2,000–2,500		
30	1,900–2,375	100–125 calories	10
40	1,800–2,250	200–250 calories	20
50	1,700–2,125	300–375 calories	30
60	1,600–2,000	400–500 calories	40
70	1,500–1,875	500–625 calories	50

* without a corresponding change in diet/activity patterns

caused by the stress/cortisol relationship rather than just by the severe diet, another study exposed a group of women to both a "stress session" and a "nonstress" (control) session on different days. The women who reacted to the stress by secreting higher levels of cortisol were the very same women who consumed more calories on the stress day compared to the low-stress day. Also of note was the fact that the women producing the most cortisol were not only hungrier, but they also showed an increase in negative moods in response to the stressors (which were significantly related to food consumption). These results suggest that stress itself, or at least the psychophysiological response to stress, can strongly influence cortisol levels and eating behavior, which, over time, could obviously have an impact on both weight and long-term health.

Okay, so now we know that the "stress" of a severe diet will make you hungry and cause you to eat more (regardless of the diet's calorie level). We also know that the stress without the diet will cause the very same thing to happen—but does this mean that *all* forms of stress will cause us to pork out? Maybe. Another study looked at a group of middle-aged men of varying socioeconomic grades (some were rich and some were poor). The fellas on the lower end of the socioeconomic ladder (the poorer guys) were significantly more likely to be overweight (visceral obesity) and to have higher cortisol values in relation to perceived stress (even though total cortisol secretion over the day of the study was not elevated). The researchers noted that the "duration of low socioeconomic conditions" (which is scientific mumbo jumbo for "being poor for a long time") seemed to worsen the effects of cortisol and strengthen the relationship between cortisol and obesity (meaning that being poor is bad for both your stress level and your waistline). Overall, the researchers concluded that the stress of a low socioeconomic status is associated with elevated cortisol secretion and with a significant, strong, and consistent relationship with obesity.

Perhaps one of the most compelling findings about the relationship between stress, cortisol, and obesity, however, comes from a study of young women by researchers at Yale University. Among these women, half of them had a high level of "cognitive dietary restraint" (meaning they put a lot of mental energy into restricting themselves from overeating and/or from certain foods). Compared to women with low levels of cognitive dietary restraint, those with high restraint scores had significantly higher cortisol levels, despite also getting more exercise (in general, moderate levels of exercise tend to reduce stress and cortisol levels). Not only have the Yale scientists shown that high levels of stress can increase cortisol levels, but they have also been at the forefront in linking those high cortisol levels to accumulation of abdominal body fat (in both men and women) and to an accelerated loss of bone mass in young and old women (more on that later).

Similar studies conducted in the Department of Neurosciences at the New Jersey Medical School used rats to investigate the relationship between stress and obesity. Results from the animal studies showed that even moderate levels of daily, unpredictable stress over the course of five weeks led to increased levels of cortisol, increased appetite and food intake, and higher body weights compared to unstressed animals. The stressed-out rats had cortisol levels that were 48 percent higher than the mellow rats, and they ate 27 percent more and became 26 percent fatter. But what does that mean for us humans? Are we destined to become fat as a result of our stressful lives? Probably—unless we learn to control the adverse effects of cortisol.

Exercise and proper diet can certainly minimize our age-related drop in metabolism and increased tendency toward weight gain, but they can also help us control our response to stress and our metabolism of cortisol. The "right" program of diet and exercise will burn calories, shed fat, relieve stress, and reduce cortisol—but most people have enough experience to show that diet and exercise have their own limitations. In fact, researchers at the University of Colorado have shown that athletes performing *too much* exercise (overtrained cross-country skiers) experience the very same adverse effects of elevated cortisol levels, such as mood disturbances, immune-system suppression, and increased levels of body fat. Of particular interest in this study was the finding that the athletes who were working out the most—those putting in the highest mileage and the longest training times—were also the ones with the highest cortisol levels, the highest body fat levels, and the poorest scores on measures of emotional outlook (more depression). Basically, they were exercising their brains out to get in better shape, but their elevated cortisol levels were hampering, and indeed outright *preventing*, their progress.

So where does this leave us? In terms of weight loss, we know quite clearly that stress, dieting, and cortisol are all detrimental to our overall goals of shedding excess body fat. We also know from decades of research that both exercise and diet can be helpful in controlling stress, cortisol, body weight, and a whole host of related health parameters. Scientists at the University of Göteborg in Sweden have shown that high cortisol levels are associated with a high waist-to-hip ratio, excess abdominal fat, elevated insulin levels, and a reduced secretion of growth hormone and testosterone—but they have also shown that a 13–14 percent reduction in cortisol levels is associated with a weight loss of more than twelve pounds. This means that despite the gloom and doom caused by the link between stress, cortisol, and obesity, we have some hope that by controlling cortisol levels we can make a positive impact on our body weight and level of body fat.

CORTISOL AND SYNDROME X

Most people have never even heard of syndrome X, which refers to a cluster of related conditions and symptoms including diabetes, insulin resistance, obesity, hypertension, high cholesterol, and heart disease (yikes!). If you are starting to gain weight, feeling low on energy, seeing your cholesterol level and blood pressure creep up, and feeling as if your mind is not quite as sharp as it used to be, then you are a likely candidate for developing (or you are already suffering from) syndrome X.

One of the key metabolic aspects of syndrome X is insulin resistance (discussed in the previous section as it relates to obesity). Insulin resistance leads to a reduction in the body's cellular response to insulin, which interferes with blood-sugar regulation, increases appetite, and blocks the body's ability to burn fat. When insulin resistance is combined with a poor diet (high in fat and/or refined carbohydrates), the result is the metabolic syndrome known as syndrome X—which can have an impact on virtually every disease process in the body.

Some authors have proposed that both insulin resistance and syndrome X are *caused* by a diet high in refined carbohydrates such as cookies, soft drinks, pasta, cereals, muffins, breads, rolls, and the like. While it is indeed true that refined carbohydrates (also known as *high-glycemic-index* carbohydrates) can raise blood levels of glucose and insulin, it is highly speculative that these junk foods actually *cause* syndrome X. (There's no controversy, however, that a diet high in such foods will certainly not help your health.) Instead, it is far more likely that the metabolic cascade of events set in motion by stress and elevated cortisol levels is the primary factor in getting a person started toward developing full-blown syndrome X—and a poor diet may hasten the trip.

People at highest risk for syndrome X are typically those of us who are approaching "middle age" (which is always a relative term). Aside from the fact that syndrome X simply leaves you feeling kind of "blah" (fatigued, fuzzy-headed, depressed, and disinterested in sex), it also sets the stage for several life-threatening conditions such as obesity, heart disease, diabetes, Alzheimer's disease, and some forms of cancer.

Among the early signs of syndrome X are low energy levels and "fuzzy" mental functioning. Very often, these feelings strike following meals, due to the body's problems handling carbohydrates. A sufferer will also notice that his clothes begin to fit a bit tighter due to a gradual weight gain of a pound or so at a time. Most problematically, the person will also have trouble *losing* those extra few pounds due to a variety of metabolic changes such as elevated blood sugar, increased insulin levels, and reduced levels of certain anabolic hormones (all of which you remember from the previous section about how stress makes us fat).

Taken separately, each of these relatively mild changes in one's metabolic machinery is not a big deal and is likely to be brushed off by the sufferer or his health-care provider with an overly simplistic recommendation to "get more exercise" or "watch what you eat." When considered *together*, however, the additive effect of each of these metabolic changes compounds a person's overall risk of serious health problems.

The primary effects of stress in raising one's risk of diabetes (only one aspect of syndrome X) are related to chronically elevated levels of glucose and insulin in the blood. Over time, elevated glucose and insulin cause body cells (primarily the ones in fat and muscle tissue) to become less sensitive to the effects of insulin, a condition known as *insulin resistance*. In response to the development of insulin resistance in these cells, the body begins to produce even more insulin—starting the vicious cycle that leads to development of full-blown diabetes.

Insulin resistance is perhaps one of the earliest metabolic events leading to full-blown syndrome X—and insulin resistance is certainly *exacerbated* by, if not exactly *caused* by, a diet high in refined carbohydrates (sugars) and by elevated cortisol levels (from chronic stress). Refined carbohydrates increase glucose and insulin levels in the blood, while cortisol reduces the effectiveness of insulin and reduces the body's ability to burn fat for energy. Both diet and exercise can play important roles in helping to control blood-sugar and insulin levels, but unless you adequately control cortisol levels, your attention to diet and exercise will have you spinning your wheels.

Adding to the complexity of the connection between stress, cortisol, and metabolic alterations such as insulin resistance is the recent finding that inadequate sleep may actually cause insulin resistance. This is particularly interesting because of the well-known link between sleep deprivation and elevated cortisol levels.

In 2001, at the Annual Scientific Meeting of the American Diabetes Association, sleep researchers from the University of Chicago presented new evidence that inadequate sleep may promote development of insulin resistance (a well-known risk factor for type-2 diabetes). The research team compared "normal" sleepers (averaging 7.5 to 8.5 hours of sleep per night) to "short" sleepers (averaging less than 6.5 hours of sleep per night), finding that the short sleepers secreted 50 percent more insulin and were 40 percent less sensitive to the effects of insulin compared to the normal sleepers. This is precisely the same effect seen during the aging process, when we begin to sleep fewer hours per night, our cortisol levels begin to rise, and our cells begin to become resistant to the effects of insulin.

Could inadequate amounts of sleep be aging us prematurely? Probably. The Chicago sleep researchers also suggested that sleep deprivation, which is becoming commonplace in industrialized countries, may play a significant role in the current epidemic of obesity and type-2 diabetes. A recent poll conducted by the National Sleep Foundation documents a steady decline in the number of hours Americans sleep each night. In 1910, the average American slept a whopping nine hours per night, in 1975, it was down to only about seven and a half hours, and today we get only about seven hours a night—and many of us get far less than that.

CORTISOL, FATIGUE, AND INSOMNIA

Mark was a building contractor who liked his job and enjoyed spending time with his family and on his hobbies (snowmobiling in winter and boating in summer). With his laid-back attitude he appeared to be about as low-stress a person as you could ever meet. Unfortunately, he often reported problems with his sleep patterns; most notably, he had great difficulty falling asleep because his mind got going "a million miles an hour" as soon as he retired for the evening. Once asleep, Mark would often wake up in the middle of the night and have trouble dropping off again. The lack of sleep was beginning to affect his work. First of all, he had a hard time getting out of bed on time in the mornings, and then once he was at work he had trouble concentrating on the precise measurements and craftsmanship necessary to do his job. How did Mark finally deal with his stress-induced insomnia and fatigue? To find out, see Chapter 10.

How do you suppose it is that stress can cause us to be fatigued during the day—but also cause us to have trouble falling asleep at night? The "dynamic duo" of chronic fatigue and insomnia would logically seem to be opposite conditions (if you're so tired, why can't you fall asleep?), but they are commonly found together in the two-thirds of the American population who report experiencing chronic stress and who get inadequate sleep. The common element? You guessed it: cortisol. Making matters worse is the fact that insomnia and fatigue often combine with each other in a vicious cycle wherein stress makes it hard to relax and fall asleep, a person's fatigued condition the next day makes stressors harder to deal with, and the additional stress causes even more difficulty falling asleep the next night. (See Figure 4.2 on the next page.)

SO WHERE DOES CORTISOL FIT IN?

As we all know by now, cortisol levels are elevated in response to stress—so any stressful events encountered in the late afternoon to early evening will hamper a person's ability to relax and fall asleep that night. If you'll recall, one of the many effects of cortisol is to increase a person's level of alertness—which is exactly what you want to avoid right before bedtime. Also, if you don't get to bed at a reasonable hour (early enough to allow a full eight to nine hours of shut-eye), your cortisol metabolism doesn't get a chance to step through its normal rhythm, which would achieve its lowest point around 2:00 A.M., as illustrated earlier. As a result, you may get only five, six, or seven hours of sleep, and you wake

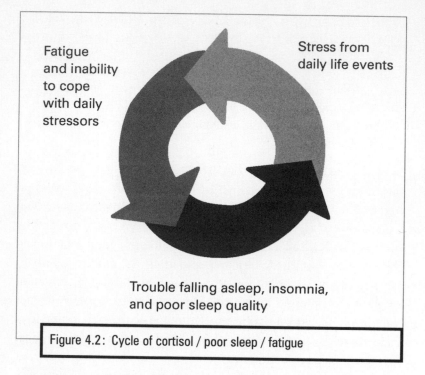

Fatigue
and inability
to cope
with daily
stressors

Stress from
daily life events

Trouble falling asleep, insomnia,
and poor sleep quality

Figure 4.2: Cycle of cortisol / poor sleep / fatigue

up groggy after having been exposed to higher than normal levels
of cortisol throughout the night.

The long-term results of sleeping less than the standard eight
hours a night most people need are annoying side effects such as
headaches, irritability, frequent infections, depression, anxiety,
confusion, and generalized mental and physical fatigue. But it's
not just that a lack of sleep leaves you feeling crappy; research
shows that even mild sleep deprivation can actually destroy one's
long-term health and increase one's risk of diabetes, obesity, and
breast cancer. In many ways, sleeping less than eight hours each
night is as bad for overall wellness as gorging on junk food or
becoming a couch potato.

Remember that cortisol levels normally peak in the early
morning (about 6:00 A.M. to 8:00 A.M.) as a way to get a person
moving and prepare her to face the challenges of the day. Between
8:00 A.M. and 11:00 A.M., cortisol levels begin to drop and gradu-

ally decline throughout the day—typically causing us to feel a drop in energy levels and ability to concentrate sometime around 3:00 P.M. to 4:00 P.M. (the "afternoon slump"). This dip in energy levels is the body's way of saying, "The day is almost over; better get ready for sleep." Unfortunately, instead of getting ready for sleep, our modern lifestyles have most of us looking for a way to boost our energy levels in the evenings so that we can get through soccer practices, piano recitals, business dinners, and time with our families. Our body clock really wants us to eat our last meal of the day around 5:00 P.M. and to be asleep by 8:00 P.M., but our wristwatch has us awake late into the night. The major problem with our modern "late to bed, early to rise" lifestyles is that our cortisol levels never have enough time to fully dissipate (which is supposed to happen overnight), so our bodies never have a chance to fully recover and repair themselves from the detrimental effects of chronic stress.

The natural rhythm of *restful* sleep follows a very specific path from the moment your head hits the pillow: breathing slows, muscles relax, heart rate and blood pressure drop, and body temperature falls. The brain releases melatonin (the "sleep hormone"), and begins its change from the rapid beta waves (indicating daytime restless wakefulness) to the slower alpha waves (indicating calm wakefulness) and eventually into the still slower theta waves that predominate during the various stages of sleep. During a full night of sleep, we normally pass through several stages of sleep: Stage 2 (lasting ten to fifteen minutes), then Stage 3 (lasting five to fifteen minutes), and finally to the deepest portion of sleep in Stage 4 (lasting about thirty minutes), and the most famous portion of the sleep cycle, REM (rapid eye movement), when we dream. This cycle, from Stage 2 to REM sleep, takes an average of ninety minutes to complete and will repeat itself over and over throughout the night. In the absence of alarm clocks, lights, and other interruptions, sleep researchers have found that the natural duration of these repeating sleep cycles (the "physiological ideal") is eight hours and fifteen minutes.

So what happens to those of us who simply can't (or won't) get that much shut-eye? Well, for one thing, blood-sugar levels will rise. Sleep researchers have shown that getting only four hours of sleep per night results in signs of impaired glucose tolerance and insulin resistance—which means that as little as a few nights of cheating on sleep can put a person in a prediabetic state. These changes in insulin action and blood-sugar control are also linked to the development of obesity. Compounding the obesity link to poor sleep is the fact that levels of both growth hormone and leptin are reduced in people who spend less time in deep sleep. Less growth hormone in the system typically means a loss of muscle and a gain of fat over time, while reduced levels of leptin will lead to hunger and carbohydrate cravings.

Let's look at the case of a typical all-American go-getter; we'll call him Driven Dan. Who's got time for sleep? Dan can't worry about the abstract risks of getting fat, developing diabetes, or contracting cancer—he has work to do, classes to take, bills to pay, soccer practices to attend, yada, yada, yada. Sound familiar? So what's the solution? Perish the thought that our friend Dan should try to do fewer things—you'll get none of that "simplify your life" stuff in this book (despite the fact that it makes perfect sense). In a perfect world, Dan may be able to work seven hours a day, enjoy a short commute to work, and have all the free time he can stand. In the real world, however (the one in which we all live), the more realistic approach for Dan (and for you?) may be to do the next best thing by getting a handle on his cortisol levels (as we'll delve into in later chapters).

CORTISOL AND SEX DRIVE

Holly and *Alan* were happily married young newlyweds with a big problem. As newlyweds, one of the things that should have held great interest for them (SEX!) offered little allure. The problem was certainly not their love and attraction for each other, but their extreme stress levels. Both Holly and Alan were (and still are) ambitious young professionals, with long stress-ful hours at the office and all the trappings of financial success (both had MBAs, drove BMWs, and lived in a beautiful home paid for by two sizable incomes). The good news is that Holly and Alan were able to reignite the spark in their love life. Learn how they did so in Chapter 8.

You don't need to read a book about the relationship between stress and disease to know that when we're stressed out we also have problems in the intimacy department. For starters, menstrual cycles get all out of whack, erections are more difficult to achieve and maintain, and overall libido (sex drive) plummets. Stress simply makes us lose interest in sex. In males, this is due primarily to a dramatic fall in testosterone levels during stressful times. In females, the stress-induced loss of sex drive is a bit more complicated, involving disruption in levels not only of testosterone, but also of estrogen, progesterone, and prolactin.

The stress/libido relationship is, predictably, tied to cortisol levels (and also to another class of chemicals from the brain—the endorphins—but more on them later). In men, elevated cortisol levels do at least a few things to suppress our sex drive. First, cortisol signals the body to reduce its production of the "prehormone" compounds that serve as the precursors to testosterone. Cut off the supply of "parts" and your production of the end product also dries up. Next, just in case any testosterone *does* get produced, cortisol also blocks the normal response of the testicles to testosterone, which is generally to make guys feel frisky. This also means that supplemental forms of testosterone, such as anabolic steroids and dietary supplements containing DHEA or androstenedione, are less likely to have any effects on libido when you're under stress. Finally, if we think for a moment about the actual mechanics of achieving an erection, it is obvious that we need a redistribution of blood flow from one place to another. When you're under stress, however, blood is being channeled to places where it can provide the most benefit—like your arms for fighting or your legs for fleeing—not to your privates.

Let's get back to the endorphins. These are the "feel-good" pain-relieving chemicals released by the brain and responsible for the euphoric feeling known as "runner's high." The interesting thing about endorphins is that they also work to suppress some of the hormonal steps leading up to testosterone production. This helps to explain the findings from studies of extreme endurance athletes wherein high levels of endorphins and cortisol are associated with low testosterone levels, reduced sperm counts, and reduced sex drive. This is not to say that aerobic exercise, such as jogging or cycling, is *bad* for you, but it emphasizes the fact that *extremes* of exercise (and inadequate recovery) are perceived by the body as stressors—and in reaction the body goes through the same stress response caused by other stressful events.

In women, the relationship between stress and reproductive function is a bit more complicated. In very basic terms, the menstrual cycle can be divided into two distinct phases. In the first phase, known as the *follicular phase*, estrogen is the dominant hormone (although there are several important hormones interacting here) and ovulation (release of an egg from the ovaries) is the primary event. The second phase of the menstrual cycle, known as the *luteal phase*, is dominated by an increase in another hormone, progesterone, which stimulates the uterus to get ready for implantation of a fertilized egg (assuming that the newly released egg meets up with an eligible sperm). Failing fertilization, the thickened uterine lining is lost in the form of blood and tissue during menstruation, and the whole cycle repeats itself in another twenty-eight days (give or take a couple days).

During stress, this extremely complex and tightly regulated hormonal balance gets all out of whack. Estrogen and progesterone levels drop (so eggs are not released from the ovaries, a condition called *anovulation*), and the uterine lining remains undeveloped (so eggs cannot be implanted). Menstrual cycles can become irregular (oligomenorrhea) or cease altogether (amenorrhea). Speaking of amenorrhea, it is interesting to note that female athletes often encounter disruptions in their menstrual cycles as a result of their

training and eating patterns. Just as with the male endurance athletes (and their low testosterone levels) mentioned above, these
female athletes tend to have low levels of estrogen and progesterone as well as a severely reduced libido. They also tend to be
dieting or at least not consuming enough calories to support the
energy demands of their sport. If you think about it, the fact that
they have no interest in sex (or the ability to get pregnant) makes
perfect sense. The change in hormone levels and the demands of
their diet and exercise regimens are being perceived by the body as
major stressors. Because the average pregnancy costs about fifty
thousand calories (and afterward another thousand calories per
day for breast-feeding), it is quite logical for the body to shut off
sexual desire (and ability) during stressful times.

So what to do? Quit your job, move to the islands, and open
up a surf shop! Your sex drive is *guaranteed* to increase. (Ever
wonder why you feel friskier when you're on vacation?—less
stress!) Not practical to move your family to Tahiti? Okay, then at
least do something about your cortisol levels. Solutions are presented in coming chapters.

CORTISOL, SUPPRESSED IMMUNE FUNCTION, AND CANCER

We know that during periods of increased stress, there is often also
an increase in the incidence of certain chronic conditions such as
asthma, allergies, and rheumatoid arthritis, as well as of gastrointestinal ailments such as irritable bowel syndrome (IBS) and
Crohn's disease. This is quite interesting, because each of these
conditions is considered to have an autoimmune component to
it—meaning that one's own immune system has gone a bit hay-
wire and has started to attack one's own tissues. In these cases,
doctors often prescribe synthetic versions of cortisol as a way to
suppress an overactive immune system, and it works quite well—
but only for a short period of time. The problem with using synthetic cortisol as a medication, however, is that too much of the

stuff, or even a modest amount for too long, leads to the very same tissue breakdown and metabolic disturbances present during chronic stress.

Medical researchers have known for more than sixty years that chronic or repeated bouts of stress will lead to a shrinking of the thymus gland (one of the key immune tissues in the body) and to a general suppression of immune-system strength. We know that cortisol has a direct effect on shrinking the thymus and inhibiting white-blood-cell production and activity. Cortisol suppresses the ability of white blood cells to secrete chemical messengers (interleukins and interferons), so the different varieties of immune-system cells are unable to communicate with each other to effectively fight off infections. Finally, and most remarkably, is the fact that cortisol can actually act as a signal to many immune-system cells to simply shut off and stop working (that is, the cells die).

Now, why would stress and cortisol have all of these detrimental effects on the immune system? You would think that during times of stress, the body would want to *increase* its resistance to invading pathogens (bacteria and viruses) rather than *decrease* this vital protection—but this is clearly not what happens.

In answering the question of why stress and cortisol would inhibit immune-system function, we need to again consider the *timing* of the stress response. Just as the relationship between cortisol and appetite has an aspect of timing to it (stress suppresses appetite for a few seconds or minutes, but then stimulates appetite for the next few hours), the relationship between cortisol and immune-system function is also mediated by timing. If we look at stress/immunity in these terms, we see that immune function is actually *stimulated* by stress for a short period of time (a few minutes). This short blast of immune-system stimulation appears to be used by the body to "wake up" existing immune-system cells as well as to "clear out" those cells that fail to work properly due to normal cell aging.

This is all very good: Now you have a short-term stressor that has ramped up immune-system activity and you're ready to fight off the invading bugs. The problem, as it has been for many of the bodily systems discussed thus far, is that a *prolonged* stress response sends these finely regulated systems into complete chaos. During periods of chronic stress, cortisol levels remain elevated and immune-system integrity begins to suffer. Not only do the chronically stimulated immune-system cells start to break down, losing their ability to fight off invading pathogens, but in some cases they can start to unleash their destructive properties on the body's own tissues, resulting in a variety of allergies, as well as in autoimmune diseases such as multiple sclerosis, lupus, fibromyalgia, and rheumatoid arthritis.

Confused yet? If not, then you should be, because most of the world's top immunologists and stress physiologists are baffled by the fact that stress increases immune-system function on the one hand, but then turns around and dismantles one of our most important protective systems on the other. One of the proposed reasons for this "Jekyll and Hyde" effect of cortisol has to do with the fact that while a stimulated immune system is good on a short-term basis, undergoing this stimulation on a long-term basis may actually lead to autoimmune diseases (wherein the immune system attacks the body's own tissues).

This makes good sense—that is, for cortisol to stimulate immune-system activity during stress, but then when cortisol levels return to normal (after the stress is over) for overall immune-system activity to do so, too. Unfortunately, our modern high-stress lifestyles (the Type C condition) don't allow cortisol levels to return to normal. Consequently, one of the body's "safety valves" comes into play, whereby chronic exposure to cortisol causes the immune-system cells to break down, thus preventing autoimmune diseases, but also reducing our ability to ward off future infections and increasing our risk for many diseases.

Speaking of autoimmune diseases, it is important to make the point (again) that glucocorticoids (of which cortisol is one) are routinely used by physicians to combat autoimmune diseases. If we think of autoimmune diseases as conditions wherein an overactive immune system attacks our joints (rheumatoid arthritis) or nerve cells (multiple sclerosis) or connective tissue (lupus), then it is logical to knock down this overzealous immune system with a huge dose of cortisol (glucocorticoids). In this way, cortisol can be thought of as being our "friend" by suppressing immune-system activity, but cortisol can also be thought of as our "enemy" because of the memory problems, muscle loss, and other side effects experienced by patients injected with high doses of glucocorticoids. Unfortunately, during times of stress these very same autoimmune diseases tend to flare up—which is confusing, because the stress-induced rise in cortisol would be expected to reduce immune-system activity and actually help control the diseases. Again, it probably comes down to timing, with short-term stress causing a temporary stimulation of immune activity and, thus, an increase in the symptoms of the autoimmune condition.

Studies in both animals and humans have noted a reduction by as much as 50 percent in levels of immune-system cells called *natural killer cells* (NK cells) following exposure to various forms of stress. NK cells typically function within the immune system to identify viruses and cancer cells. In one study of breast cancer patients, the level of emotional stress caused by the initial cancer diagnosis was directly related to NK cell activity. In these women, a higher stress level predicted a reduced ability of NK cells to destroy cancer cells as well as a poorer response to interventions aimed at improving NK cell activity. From animal studies, we know that cortisol not only suppresses the number and activity of these NK cells, but also promotes the synthesis of new blood vessels in tumors (a process called *angiogenesis*) and accelerates the growth of certain kinds of tumors. The bottom line here may be that chronic stress can accelerate the growth of cancer cells in the body as well as block the body's ability to battle the disease.

Heightened stress levels have also been linked to adverse effects on the balance of intestinal microflora, which are known to respond to changes in both diet and stress level. These beneficial bacteria live in our intestinal tract, and while they are intimately

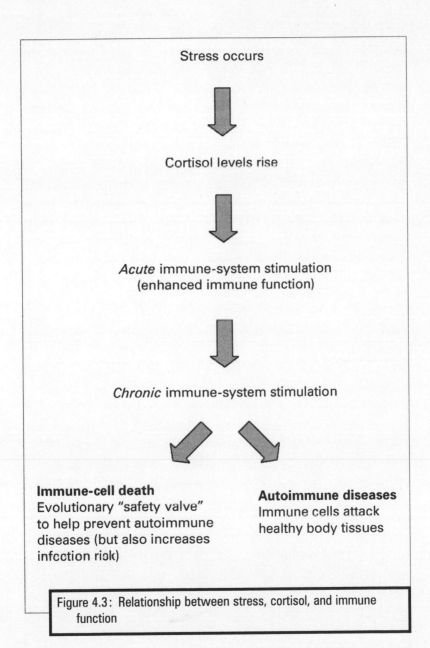

Figure 4.3: Relationship between stress, cortisol, and immune function

involved with optimal gastrointestinal function (more on that later), they also play a vital role in helping to support immune function. In a study of fighter pilots preparing for simulated battle (a fairly stressful event), distinct reductions were noted in the numbers of "good" bacteria (lactobacilli and bifidobacteria), along with a corresponding increase in the numbers of "bad" bacteria (*E. coli*, enterobacteria, and clostridia). The outcome for these pilots was, predictably, a sharp increase in their reported incidence of sore throats, headaches, colds, diarrhea, and upset stomachs.

Numerous studies in animals and humans have shown that both acute and chronic stress increases susceptibility to infectious diseases. In particular, the risk of upper-respiratory-tract infections (URTIs) is sharply increased, so that people who are under the greatest stress (or who deal with it poorly) are the ones who most often get sick. Students catch colds during exam week, and accountants get sore throats in April, when they're filing dozens of last-minute tax returns.

So, after all this discussion about the suppression of immune-system function by stress, who do you think gets sick most often?

In some stress-management clinics, the primary determinants of whether or not a given person will get sick include:

- the number of major life events in past year (divorce, death in the family, change in job or location, etc.)

- a psychological perception that daily demands exceed coping resources and/or support system

- current emotional state

Of this short list of three "sickness determinants," researchers have found that the overall degree of psychological stress is strongly related, in a dose-response fashion, to URTIs (upper-respiratory-tract infections) and other breakdowns in immune-system integrity (such as gastrointestinal health). This means the more stressed out you are, the more likely you are to get sick.

What demographic group, among all others, suffers from the highest degree of stress-related disease?

- Wealthy investment bankers? No.

- Stressed-out college students? No.

- Single mothers working two jobs and driving beat-up 1975 Chevy Chevettes? Yes!

The most direct example of the chronically elevated human stress response can be observed every day in the lives of a large part of the American (and worldwide) population. These are the folks who are driving a junker car (and hoping it makes it) to their second job. They are hoping the money from that second paycheck will last to the end of the month when the bills are due. They are *not* the people whom you see commiserating with each other about their terrible jobs on sitcoms such as *Friends*. The constant unrelenting stress of making ends meet, job instability, sleep deprivation, poor diet, lack of outlets for stress, and overall lack of control combine to increase the risk of disease by a factor of five to ten times!

Unfortunately, none of the information or recommendations that follow in this book will alleviate the actual stressors encountered by the "working poor" or by the "working middle class" (wherever you choose to draw the economic line)—but much of what follows can be used to reduce the damage wreaked by stress on all of us.

CORTISOL AND CARDIOVASCULAR DISEASE

A large and exceedingly important part of the stress response is its direct and rapid effect on the cardiovascular system. As outlined previously, the fight-or-flight response is meant to prepare your body for forceful physical activity—but no matter whether you're saved by your fists (fight) or your feet (flight), your cardiovascular system had better be ready to support whatever vigorous activity you decide to undertake. This means ramping up heart rate, blood pressure, and cardiac output (the amount of blood your heart pumps). It also means shutting down certain nonessential uses of blood (such as digestion) and shunting that blood to more important areas—like the arms and legs, where it can fuel the fighting/ fleeing muscles. Shunting blood all around the body means coordinating the dilation (relaxation) of some blood vessels and the constriction (narrowing) of others, an effect that results in elevated blood pressure during periods of stress.

What a great set of effects! If you were a race car, this stress-induced series of events would be analogous to a supercharger, and—ZOOM!—away you'd race. The key problem may already be apparent to you: Keep that supercharger opened full throttle for too long, or use it too frequently, and you're likely to blow a gasket, throw a piston, or destroy the entire engine. What this means for your heart and cardiovascular system is clear: Chronic activation of your stress-response system increases your risk of blowing a gasket in your heart (otherwise known as heart disease).

We know that elevated blood pressure can accelerate damage to the interior lining of blood vessels. These small areas of vessel damage become perfect "docking points" for circulating particles of sugar, fat, and cholesterol—so there they stick (and stress has already elevated each of them to serve as fuel for your expected fight/flight). As if that weren't already bad enough, your blood gets thicker because of the tendency of stress hormones to promote blood clotting. Thick blood might be a good thing if you come out on the losing side of a fight, but it's not a good thing if you're simply sitting in a traffic jam with a rapid heart rate, elevated blood pressure, and constricted blood vessels.

A variety of animal studies (in monkeys, rats, mice, and dogs) has supported the concept that stress leads to heart disease. Across these studies, it is clear that the animals subjected to the most social stress are also the ones that develop the most or worst blockages in their blood vessels. High-fat diets appear to compound the problems (duh!). Interestingly, physical stressors do not seem to be quite as bad for the heart—probably because running around, wrestling, or fighting appear to help dissipate stress hormones.

Health professionals have known for decades that blood pressure, cholesterol levels, heart attacks, and strokes are closely related to overall degree of stress. Emotional state has been known to trigger heart attacks in many people, with feelings of sadness, anger, and "control" (that is, how much control people feel they have over their lives and/or destinies) being linked to causation of heart disease. Overall, risk for coronary heart disease is three to five times greater in people with higher levels of anger, anxiety, and worry compared to people who report lower levels.

Researchers from the Mayo Clinic have shown that psychological stress is one of the strongest risk factors for heart attacks. Furthermore, when calculating the economic costs of a high-stress lifestyle, economists have shown that hospital usage costs more than $9,500 per visit in heart-attack patients with high stress, but just over $2,100 in those with low stress.

Most of us understand that heart disease is the leading cause of death in the United States and much of the Western world. Almost all cases of heart attack and stroke are due to atherosclerosis caused by high blood pressure, high cholesterol, diabetes (high blood-sugar and insulin levels), smoking, and physical inactivity. What many people fail to realize, however, is that the cardiovascular aspects of heightened stress may merely be the tip of the iceberg when it comes to the long-term health consequences of elevated cortisol levels.

The good news is that there also appears to be a powerful inverse relationship between stress and the strength of one's social network—meaning that strong social support (from friends, family, and coworkers) can be a key factor in reducing the link between stress and heart disease. Stated another way, those with a stronger social network can withstand more stress before succumbing to disease. More good news is found in reports of the association between stress and hypertension: The dissipation of

stress, through either meditation or exercise, helps to bring blood
pressure back to normal levels.

YOUR BRAIN ON CORTISOL: ANXIETY, DEPRESSION, AND ALZHEIMER'S DISEASE

Rachel was a single mom with two young children. In addition
to her full-time job at her daughter's day care, she also volun-
teered as a chaperone for her son's Boy Scout troop. As you
can imagine, Rachel had more than enough stress in her life in
the form of financial constraints, child-care issues, and being a
single parent. As a result, she often felt her patience wear thin,
especially when confronted with a dozen screaming Boy
Scouts at the end of a stressful day at the day care. Take a look
at Chapter 8 to see how Rachel used specific nutritional supplements to deal with heightened anxiety and irritability.

Who among us is not affected to some degree by periods of stress
and anxiety? For virtually everybody, modern lifestyles create a fair
amount of tension, irritability, worry, and frustration, which can
lead to feelings of chronic anxiety and depression. In fact, some-
where between 5 and 20 percent of Americans will experience
depression severe enough to warrant medication or other therapy.

In addition to the emotional effects brought on by chronic
stress are its direct effects on the brain. Research has shown that
stress can increase the incidence of simple forgetfulness and accelerate the development of full-blown memory loss and Alzheimer's
disease. Each of these conditions involves a degree of mental deterioration characterized by damage to and the death of nerve cells
in the brain—and it has been estimated that as many as 30 to 50
percent of adults in industrialized countries suffer from these conditions.

The changes in mood that accompany periods of heightened
stress also bring reduced energy levels, feelings of fatigue, irritability, inability to concentrate, and feelings of depression—all

of which are related to the same class of brain chemicals, called *neurotransmitters*. Most notable (and scary), perhaps, are the findings that chronic stress can lead to actual *physical* changes in the arrangement of the neurons (nerve cells) in the brain. In other words, we're talking now about stress changing both the function and the *shape* of your brain. No wonder it doesn't work the way it's supposed to!

Related to depression, but different in a number of ways, is anxiety—that nagging, sometimes overwhelming, sense of disquiet or unease that most of us experience to one degree or another at least occasionally. Anxiety can get out of hand in the form of panic attacks or obsessive-compulsive disorder, both of which appear to be associated with a chronically overactive stress response (especially with elevated catecholamines, that is, epinephrine and norepinephrine).

Several anxiety disorders exist, many of which are typically combined with other emotional disorders, such as depression. The overall severity of the various anxiety disorders can be thought of as existing on a continuum, with a given individual experiencing mild cases of multiple types of anxiety disorders or a more severe case of a specific anxiety disorder. The most common anxiety-related conditions are panic disorder and obsessive-compulsive disorder, and both are related to the overall magnitude of the stress response and cortisol production.

Panic disorder occurs in approximately 1 to 2 percent of the population. It typically begins in young adulthood, and women are twice as likely as men to suffer from it. The condition manifests itself in episodes of extreme anxiety and fear. These panic attacks, as they are commonly known, can last from a few seconds to a few hours, and may include real physical symptoms such as shortness of breath, sweating, irregular heartbeat, dizziness, and faintness. They can be so severe that the sufferer ends up in the emergency room with fears that she or he is having a heart attack. Compounding this condition is the anticipatory anxiety that plagues the sufferer after experiencing these attacks, leading to a vicious cycle in which more anxiety is caused by worrying about having future panic attacks. It is unclear in these situations whether elevated cortisol levels are the primary causative factor that *induces* the panic attacks, or whether high cortisol levels *result from* the initial panic attack and, while remaining elevated, exacerbate the condition and set the stage for another attack.

Another variant of anxiety is obsessive-compulsive disorder (OCD), which produces obsessive, almost inescapable thoughts and compulsive behaviors the sufferer cannot help but perform. About 2 percent of the population suffers from OCD. Females are slightly more susceptible than males, and, as with panic disorder, it typically first manifests in young adulthood. People with OCD are in a sense better adapted to anxiety than are individuals with panic disorder, because those with OCD avoid panic attacks via their compulsive behaviors, which may act in a way as "destress" exercises. Unfortunately, the behaviors or rituals needed to satisfy the compulsion often interfere with normal activities and relationships. Most of the compulsions fall into one of four categories, including checking, cleaning, counting, and avoidance. In many cases, it is thought that these compulsions act as simple defense mechanisms, whereby the compulsive behavior or obsessive thought patterns help to reduce feelings of anxiety. However, these thoughts and behaviors become ritualized and inescapable, leading to a heightened level of stress and anxiety as they begin to disrupt activities of daily living. Treatment for OCD generally involves both behavioral therapy and drug treatment, but the disorder often persists over time unless the root cause of the stress is fully addressed.

Clearly, various treatments exist for people suffering from anxiety. Aside from behavioral therapy, which is often all that is needed (especially for simple phobias), several medicinal treatments exist that vary according to the type of anxiety and whether or not the anxiety is combined with other problems. Traditional tranquilizers, such as Valium, are often the first medications that come to mind. However, anxiety frequently goes hand in hand with depression, and antidepressants such as Prozac, Zoloft, and Wellbutrin are often prescribed to treat the combination of problems. For individuals who prefer a more "natural" approach to treatment, there are many alternatives in the form of supplements, herbs, and combination products that may help alleviate anxiety, reduce stress, and control cortisol levels. These are covered in detail in upcoming chapters.

The ultimate cause of depression is exceedingly complex—and well beyond the scope of this book. From our perspective relating to the association of stress with depression, however, it is known that cortisol levels tend to be higher in people suffering from depression, while levels of brain neurotransmitters such as dopamine, norepinephrine, and serotonin are lower. Does this mean that cortisol lowers brain neurotransmitters or causes depression? Not necessarily, but we know quite clearly that the people who are under the highest levels of stress also tend to be the ones who succumb to periods of moderate depression. Part of the reason may be that during periods of heightened stress, the brain becomes accustomed to high cortisol levels, and when the stressor is removed (or reduced) the brain is unable to function effectively. We know from animal studies, for example, that the brains of rats exposed to repeated stresses eventually become resistant to specific pleasure pathways—so higher and higher levels of the brain's "feel-good" chemicals (dopamine, serotonin, and endorphins) are needed to induce a response. It has also been known for more than twenty years that patients given high doses of cortisol-like drugs (such as corticosteroids to treat autoimmune diseases) also tend to develop memory problems and signs of clinical depression.

So, in asking ourselves the question "Does cortisol cause depression?"—the answer is definitely, probably "maybe." It certainly appears that having elevated cortisol levels raises one's risk of developing depression. It also appears that cortisol does a pretty good job of gumming up the works when it comes to the synthesis, transport, breakdown, and overall activity of the neurotransmitters in the brain. Finally, we also know that using specialized drugs to "shut off" the production of cortisol can reduce the symptoms of depression—but these drugs, known as *adrenal steroidogenesis inhibitors*, have a list of nasty side effects as long as your arm.

Again, however, if we look at the relationship between stress and brain function, we see a two-phase effect, wherein short-term stress appears to enhance cognitive function, while chronic stress disrupts many aspects of brain neurochemistry. Researchers theorize that it works something like this: Acute stress causes an increase in blood flow, oxygen, and glucose to the muscles (for fight/flight), and also to the brain. We know that hypoglycemia (low blood sugar) can impair concentration and ability to think, so the increased supply of glucose should, at least transiently, increase brain power. And it does; studies of people exposed to short-term stressors show that they have an enhanced memory capacity and ability for problem solving. Unfortunately, the brain-boosting effects of stress are short-lived (lasting less than thirty minutes), because then the body is awash in cortisol, which causes blood flow and glucose delivery to the brain to fall. Prolonged exposure of brain cells (neurons) to cortisol reduces their ability to take up glucose (their only fuel source) and—here's the really scary part—causes them to shrink in size! So there you have it: Repeated stress and prolonged exposure to cortisol—once again, the Type C condition—actually lead to a progressive destruction of the neurons in the brain. Not good.

It is important to note that while it is quite tempting to make the obvious link between cortisol levels and Alzheimer's disease, we simply have no *direct* evidence that cortisol *causes* Alzheimer's disease, although chronic stress and elevated cortisol levels certainly appear able to make the situation much worse. It is true that most of us past the age of forty will begin to experience some degree of "normal" age-related memory loss (often called *age-related cognitive decline* or ARCD), but this is a far cry from the severe mental deterioration (senile dementia) usually seen with Alzheimer's disease. Although Alzheimer's disease may affect as many as 50 percent of people over eighty-five years old to a certain degree, the condition is a whole lot more than simple forgetfulness. Studies of the brain neurons from Alzheimer's patients show a clear pattern of death and destruction in the parts of the brain involved in memory and higher thoughts.

It is also interesting, in light of our discussions of depression and anxiety, to note that Alzheimer's disease often begins with damage to the brain cells that produce a neurotransmitter called *acetylcholine*. This loss of acetylcholine causes symptoms ranging from the subtle, such as trouble remembering names or dates, to the more noticeable behavioral problems, such as depression and anxiety, and eventually to disorientation and a loss of ability care for oneself. Drug treatment with Cognex or Aricept (which increase acetylcholine action) can produce a modest improvement in mild cases of Alzheimer's disease, but no existing drugs are able to restore normal function to the damaged regions of the brain.

So, stress and cortisol are erasing your memory, dashing your emotions, causing you anxiety, and killing your brain cells. Yikes! But you can do something about it. There are lots of steps you can take to make positive impacts on your stress response, on your level of cortisol, and on your feelings of depression and anxiety. That's what the next several chapters are about.

CORTISOL AND YOUR GUT

The image of stress-induced ulcers has been with us for decades. You've probably seen, on a TV sitcom or other such venue, the stereotypical portrayal of the stressed-out executive. Deadlines loom, stress builds, and the businessman gulps down antacids to quell the burning ulcer in his stomach. Far from being one of the many Hollywood overexaggerations, the phenomenon of stress-induced ulcers and other digestive problems has been documented in the medical literature for more than fifty years. From a physiological point of view, we know quite clearly that any stressful event will cause digestion to cease. Blood flow is diverted from the digestive organs to the heart and muscles, secretion of saliva and digestive enzymes is slowed, and intestinal contractions and absorption of nutrients stop. This rapid shutdown of the digestive process makes perfect sense, because from the standpoint of long-term survival it is more important to get away from the dangerous stressor (the lion) than to fully digest all your food. There will be plenty of time for digestion later; right now you need to save your skin. It is interesting to note, however, that even while stress hormones are signaling the body to shut down digestion, these same hormones, when kept elevated for more than a few minutes, are telling us to eat—and eat a lot!

Medical evidence shows quite clearly that ulcers of the stomach (gastric ulcers) and intestine (duodenal ulcers) are much more common in people who are anxious, depressed, or under chronic or repeated stress. In these situations, which are all examples of chronic stressors, many of the digestive actions are curtailed, so the body also backs off on its production of protective measures—such as the mucus that lines the stomach, and the bicarbonate that counteracts the highly acidic gastric juices. Sounds logical, right? And it is. Why have the body taking a lot of protective measures against acid that will never be secreted (because you're under stress)? The problems start to occur when a person experiences the repeated cycles of high stress followed by low/normal stress that have become commonplace in our modern society. This sets up the digestive system for total confusion. Most of the time the body won't be able to secrete enough digestive enzymes to properly digest food (producing nausea, constipation, gas, and bloating). During the "lucky" times when a body *can* secrete enough digestive enzymes to properly break down food, the protective mechanisms are far from fully operational—which puts a person at risk for damage to her gastrointestinal tract (because the enzymes digest the gut's lining in addition to digesting the food). This scenario says a lot about why several bouts of stress are known to cause more ulcers than a longer continuous period of heightened stress.

To compound the problem, other factors, such as immune-system function and the body's control of inflammation and wound healing, come into play. It is well described in the medical literature that both repeated periods of acute stress and continuous periods of chronic stress are associated with suppressed immune-system activity. This has a direct bearing on ulcer development, because less immune-system activity means more growth and higher activity of a bacterium called *Heliobacter pylori*, which infects the stomach and causes ulcers in 80 percent of the people infected with it. Topping off the tissue damage caused by the accelerated growth of *H. pylori* is a suppression of the body's ability to heal that damage because of an inhibition in prostaglandin synthesis. Prostaglandins are typically produced in response to tissue damage, where they help reduce inflammation and accelerate healing. During times of stress, however, the synthesis of prostaglandins is curtailed, which suggests that stress not only increases the rate at which ulcers may form, but also slows the rate at which they are repaired.

Aside from ulcers, the most common stress-related gut disease may be irritable bowel syndrome (IBS)—and most of us will experience some degree of IBS during our lifetime. The term *IBS* is really a catchall name for a variety of intestinal disorders, including colitis (inflammation of the lining of the large intestine, also known as the colon), in which abdominal pain is accompanied by diarrhea and/or constipation, bloating, gas, and, occasionally, passing of mucus or blood. The majority of the gastrointestinal conditions falling under the IBS umbrella are either caused by or exacerbated by periods of heightened stress.

So, again, we have bad news about stress and cortisol for an important body system. Stress leads to poor digestion, ulcerated stomachs, and inflamed intestines—not a pretty picture. These effects tend to result in poor dietary choices, suboptimal nutritional status, and the logical drop in energy levels and overall feelings of well-being. Getting stress and cortisol levels under control can help to reverse these problems.

CORTISOL, CONNECTIVE TISSUE, OSTEOPOROSIS, AND ARTHRITIS

Aging, as most of us know all too well, is associated with dramatic changes in some of the structural aspects of our bodies—areas such as bone and muscle strength, skin elasticity, and joint function. Profound changes in body composition also accompany advancing age, so we progressively gain fat, but lose muscle (sarcopenia), bone (osteopenia/osteoporosis), and joint cartilage (arthropenia/arthritis). This means we are likely to get weaker (due to having less muscle), feel tired (due to reduced aerobic endurance), and lose our ability to get around efficiently. Many people simply accept these changes as inevitable effects of the normal aging process—but they're not.

Luckily, researchers are learning more and more about the precise causes of age-related losses in connective tissues (muscle, bone, cartilage, skin, hair, and nails). While the aging of these tissues remains quite complex, scientists are narrowing down the list of potential mediating factors—and once again elevated cortisol levels are implicated as one of the primary markers for accelerating these tissue losses (along with low levels of anabolic hormones such as estrogen in women and testosterone and DHEA in men).

Also fortunate is the fact that age-related loss of connective tissue can be reversed, even in individuals nearing a hundred years of age. Regular exercise programs incorporating strength training, with or without aerobic exercise, have been shown to preserve or increase amounts of muscle, bone, and cartilage in older adults, while also improving independence. In addition, dietary factors such as maintaining a protein intake of about one gram of protein per pound of body weight and a calcium intake of at least fifteen hundred milligrams per day are well known to lead to positive benefits in terms of maintaining muscle and bone mass with age.

The relationship between elevated cortisol levels and an accelerated loss of cartilage, bone, and muscle has been demonstrated in numerous situations, including cases of people with Cushing's syndrome (where elevated cortisol results in severe osteoporosis and arthritis) and anorexia nervosa (where elevated cortisol leads to bone and muscle loss). Studies such as these have also determined that curing the diseases, and thereby removing the source of excess cortisol production, also restores cartilage, bone, and muscle tissues. In experimental studies, cortisol has been shown to decrease levels of connective-tissue growth factors and inhibit the activity of bone-building cells (osteoblasts), muscle-building cells (satellite cells), and cartilage-building cells (chondrocytes). So here we have a situation in which excess cortisol levels not only accelerate the breakdown of connective tissues, but also interfere with the biochemical process of building and repairing those same tissues.

The same scenario of increased loss and suppressed repair is seen in related connective tissues—such as skin, hair, and nails. The actions of cortisol to enhance catabolism (breakdown) of many forms of connective tissues (of which skin, hair, and nails are a form) are well documented in the medical literature, and while these problems may not be of the same health magnitude as osteoporosis, nobody wants to have dry skin, thin hair, and cracked fingernails.

Most of us who have passed the age of forty have probably begun losing substantial amounts of muscle, bone, and cartilage—and our skin is a far cry from the soft, smooth stuff we were born with. We start to see these declines in connective-tissue quantity and quality starting in our mid-thirties and early forties, and by the time we're in our seventies, we're down about 20 percent from where we were in our twenties. These losses have all sorts of implications for how strong we are, how many calories we burn, how much energy we have, how we feel, and how we look. Elevated levels of cortisol as we age have been implicated in the acceleration of connective-tissue destruction, while declining levels of estrogen (in women), testosterone (in men), and IGF-1 and growth hormone (in both sexes) are known to be part of our hampered ability to rebuild the damaged tissue.

The good news (for connective-tissue maintenance) is that a series of studies conducted at Tufts University and Penn State

University have shown dramatic benefits in countering the frailty that is associated with extreme muscle, cartilage, and bone loss in the elderly. Results from these studies show that frail elderly participants are able to increase muscle and bone mass and *double* their muscle strength and power with resistance training performed two to three times a week. Participants in the exercise programs were able to get around more easily and with less joint pain than they could prior to the training. An interesting side benefit of the added muscle was an average 15 percent increase in daily caloric expenditure when compared to sedentary volunteers.

It's a bit harder to assess the effects of elevated cortisol levels on other connective tissues in humans, such as skin, hair, and nails. However, laboratory studies have shed some interesting light on the fact that excess cortisol bears a wide range of adverse effects on the underlying biochemistry of the skin and related tissues. For example, researchers from Finland have shown that while a low level of cortisol is able to stimulate the synthesis and slow the breakdown (by about 25 percent) of structural skin elements such as hyaluronan and proteoglycans, higher levels of cortisol have exactly the opposite effect, reducing synthesis and accelerating degradation of these compounds by more than 40 percent. Both hyaluronan and proteoglycans are responsible for hydrating the skin by attracting and holding adequate amounts of moisture—so reduced levels of these compounds in the skin mean that the skin dries out. Similar effects have been noted for related skin proteins, such as elastin (needed for skin elasticity) and collagen (needed for skin strength), and have led many researchers to hypothesize that elevated cortisol levels may be responsible for accelerated skin "aging" and the overall skin atrophy (wrinkling) observed during drug treatment with synthetic cortisol.

CORTISOL AND AGING

Although you can't do anything about your age, it is probably important to discuss the differences in stress response between younger and older people. In very general terms, it appears to be true that as we age, we become less able to deal effectively with stress. This means that for the same "load" of stress, whether from exercise, illness, emotions, or whatever, a younger person will tend to "deal better" with the stressor compared to an older person. The primary difference does not seem to be much of a difference in the initial response to the stressor; old folks tend to secrete just as many stress hormones as their younger counterparts (though older folks also tend to have higher cortisol levels even under normal, nonstressed conditions). Instead, younger subjects tend to recover faster from stress, so they're able to get their cortisol levels back to within normal ranges in a much shorter period of time compared to older subjects. Being able to quickly turn off the stress response following a given stressor also appears to be associated with a slower growth of cancer cells (tumors), so the youngsters appear have the edge when it comes to fending off cancer (at least in lab rats).

To better understand the relationship between cortisol and aging, let's consider the situation of the salmon. You probably know the basics of the story: The salmon swims upstream for thousands of miles, spawns, and quickly dies. (Some life!) If you were to catch a salmon right after spawning, you'd see a few interesting things, such as a poor immune system, lots of infections, unhealed wounds, stomach ulcers, etc. Sounds like an overactive stress response—and that's exactly what it is. Marine biologists have studied the physiology of spawning salmons to find that, lo and behold, they have outrageously high cortisol levels. Take it one step further and remove the adrenal glands from these salmon, and guess what happens? Having no adrenal glands means that the salmon has no cortisol secretion and no rapid death; they live on perfectly well for another year or so (which is quite a long time for a fish). The primary reason for cortisol levels to go completely crazy in salmon is that they rapidly develop an inability to regulate their cortisol secretion. For some reason, their bodies fail to recognize the fact that they have plenty of cortisol in their system, so the adrenals just keep churning out more and more—and every organ system rapidly deteriorates. A similar age-related breakdown in the regulation of cortisol secretion occurs in other animals, including mice, rats, dogs, monkeys, baboons, and humans (though none quite as dramatically as in the salmon).

So does this mean we're all destined to succumb to cortisol-related organ failure as we age? Certainly not. Making some of the right choices in terms of exercise regimen, dietary intake, sleep patterns, and judicious use of nutritional supplements can go a long way toward retarding some of what we now view as "age-related" changes in how our bodies work and how we look and feel.

Summary

Whew! If the preceding information doesn't stress you out (even a little bit) then you haven't been reading very closely. At first glance, many of us might view the close relationship between stress, cortisol, and the long list of chronic diseases as a hopeless disaster just waiting to happen—and for a great many people, it is. The good news, however, is that armed with the right information and the proper motivation, one can do a great deal to counteract these potential problems. The general idea is to control the stress response in such a way that cortisol levels are maintained within their optimal range—not too high and not too low—with long-term health and wellness as the outcome. The rest of the book shows you how.

CHAPTER 5

Counteracting the Effects of Chronic Stress

A sk almost anybody about their stress level and you're bound to hear that it's high (unless you tend to surround yourself with Type B laid-back folks, like Californian surfers). Enduring a high level of stress is almost a badge of honor these days; if you don't claim to be under extreme stress, then you might feel that others will view you as somewhat of a slacker.

Okay, so let's accept the fact that most of us have plenty of stress to deal with. Is this necessarily a bad thing? No, because some people can handle a great deal of stress without succumbing to any of its detrimental health effects. Some people even claim to thrive on stress, when we know that what they really thrive on is the jolt of adrenaline and endorphins stressful situations cause their bodies to produce. Unfortunately, while adrenaline and endorphins will certainly leave us pumped up with energy and good feelings (at least for a few minutes), the resulting cortisol secretion can get us into health trouble over the long term.

But how do you know if all this applies to you? How do you know where you fall on the stress spectrum? How do you know if you're at risk for all the nasty health problems outlined in the preceding four chapters? Simple. Refer back to the results of your

Stress Self-Test, from the Preface. (If you haven't yet taken the test, totaled your results, and discovered your cortisol index, now is a good time to take a few minutes and do so.) Chances are, you're a Stressed Jess. That means everything included in this book—from the warnings about the effects of excessive stress and increased cortisol levels, to the advice about how you can counteract those effects—applies to you.

But even if you're not always a Stressed Jess, there are almost certainly times when a Strained Jane or a Relaxed Jack could use a helping hand with stress management. Whether you're a hard-charging Type A go-getter or a more relaxed, roll-with-the-punches Type B, we are all periodically at risk for slipping into the Type C lifestyle (characterized by elevated cortisol levels). For those Janes and Jacks out there, this book can be used as an a la carte resource; try a bit of this and a little of that to see which cortisol-control strategies work most effectively for your particular situation.

ADRENAL STRESS-TESTING KITS

Should you run out and purchase one of those at-home kits that measure cortisol levels in saliva or urine? Probably not. Although quite a cottage industry has sprung up to sell you at-home hormone-testing kits, the validity and utility of such kits are limited—and the same goes for the more sophisticated hormone analysis that can be ordered by your doctor. Why? The main reason these tests are unnecessary for most people is because levels of cortisol, DHEA, and related hormones fluctuate normally throughout the day and can change at a moment's notice. This means that the very act of taking the test is likely to change the results, making them virtually useless unless administered in just the right way, which is very difficult even under controlled laboratory conditions.

In most cases, however, you'll already know whether you're experiencing heightened stress. By answering the questions in the Stress Self-Test, you can get a very good idea of how much stress you're exposed to, how you tend to deal with that stress, and what level of risk that stress may pose for your long-term health. (You'll also save yourself the $70 to $380 that is typically charged for the mail-order adrenal stress tests.)

CONTROLLING THE STRESS RESPONSE: THE SENSE PROGRAM

Some of the best news contained in this book is the fact that there are almost as many different ways to *deal* with stress as there are things that *cause* stress. We all know the basics for coping with stress (Grandma has been telling us for years), but we often forget just how effective some of those simple remedies really can be. Perhaps the most effective antistress activities are also the easiest to accomplish; practices such as eating a balanced diet, getting adequate rest, and performing some regular exercise can do wonders for helping the body adapt and respond to stressful events. Unfortunately, stress often causes us to do just the opposite in each of these areas; we eat junk, we can't seem to relax, and we have no time for exercise, each of which only serves to compound the problem and exacerbate the detrimental effects of stress on our bodies. Controlling your individual stress response with various relaxation techniques can help to modulate cortisol secretion and normalize metabolism, but for many people such techniques simply are unrealistic in the face of their hectic lifestyles. So what to do?

We already know from the preceding chapters that controlling cortisol levels will yield all sorts of wonderful health benefits. Returning cortisol to a normal range will bring caloric expenditure back to normal levels, reduce body-fat levels, preserve muscle mass, decrease appetite, and increase energy levels and that's just some of the effects you'll be able to *feel*. Other benefits of controlling cortisol levels, such as reducing cholesterol and blood sugar, maintaining brain power, reducing bone loss, and strengthening immune function, will occur more "silently"—meaning you're still reaping the benefits but you won't necessarily notice them in the same way as you will an increased energy level or a slimmer waistline.

To reduce the incidence of certain diseases, the use of behavioral interventions that reduce stress can be just as beneficial for long-term health as can quitting smoking, losing weight, reducing cholesterol levels, eating well, or exercising. In other words, if it's possible to avoid stressful situations, then that is the obvious first course of action. Unfortunately, avoiding stress is not always possible or realistic for most of us. Therefore, either you need to learn how to deal with stress as effectively as possible—often referred to as *stress management*—or you need to find a way to reduce the effects of stress on your body.

The question, of course, is deciding on the best approach to controlling cortisol levels for *you*. For some people, a stress-management approach such as relaxation techniques is the most appropriate method of controlling cortisol, while others may prefer to exercise their cortisol levels into normal ranges, and still others may turn to dietary supplements as a convenient way to get cortisol levels under control.

The sections that follow summarize a program of general recommendations for controlling cortisol levels. This approach is called the SENSE program. SENSE stands for **S**tress management, **E**xercise, **N**utrition, **S**upplements, and **E**valuation —the five key areas that can be readily acted upon by anyone to control cortisol levels. (For more detailed coverage of the topics of diet, exercise, relax-

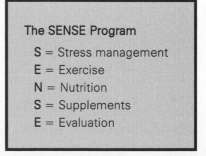

The SENSE Program
S = Stress management
E = Exercise
N = Nutrition
S = Supplements
E = Evaluation

ation, and other stress-management techniques, numerous excellent books are available; see the Resources section in the back of this book for some recommendations. See also Chapter 12, devoted entirely to the SENSE program.)

STRESS MANAGEMENT AND AVOIDANCE

Ideas and theories abound for the management of stress and the modulation of the stress response. Many of these ideas revolve around some aspect of regaining "control" over the stress response, typically by attempting to control the degree of stress or make the stressor occur with predictability. Why should this make any difference—after all, a stressor is a stressor, right? Maybe not. For example, *any* lion charging at you from the bushes is going to be stressful, but knowing *where* and *when* that lion will charge may make the stress a bit more manageable.

We know from studies of both animals and humans that at least three factors can make a huge difference in how the body responds to a given stressor: whether there is any *outlet* for the stress, whether the stressor is *predictable*, and whether the human or animal thinks they have any *control* over the stressor. These three factors—outlet, predictability, and control—emerge as modulating factors again and again in research studies of stress. For example, put a rat in a cage and subject it to a series of low-voltage electric shocks (sounds pretty stressful), and the rat gets elevated cortisol levels and develops ulcers (you would too). Take another rat, give it the same series of shocks, but also give it an outlet for its stress—such as something to chew on, something to eat, or a wheel to run on—and its cortisol levels do not go up (as much) and it does not get ulcers. The same is true for humans under stress: Go for a run, scream at the wall, or do something else that serves as an outlet for controlling cortisol levels—and cortisol levels are reduced (somewhat) and many of the detrimental effects of stress are counteracted (or at least modulated).

Let's turn now to the second of the three stress modulators, predictability. Let's say that somebody woke you up in the middle of the night, put you on a plane, and then made you jump out of it at ten thousand feet. Pretty stressful, huh? This experience would certainly be accompanied by elevated heart rate and blood pressure, changes in blood levels of glucose and fatty acids, and, of course, a huge increase in blood cortisol levels. What do you think would happen if you were forced to do this every other night or so for the next few months? Far from being a stressed-out bundle of nerves, you would actually get accustomed to it—and your stress response would become less pronounced. This scenario has actually been studied in army rangers training at jump school to become paratroopers. At the start of training, the soldiers underwent enormous increases in cortisol levels during each jump, but by the end of the course, their stress responses were virtually nonexistent. By making the stressor more predictable, the stress response of each soldier was controlled to a much greater degree (though skydiving will probably never become a completely stress-free activity).

Finally, the concept of *control* is central to understanding why some people respond to a stressor with gigantic elevations in cortisol, while other people respond to the same stressor with a much lower cortisol response. This idea has been demonstrated in rats that have been trained to press a lever to avoid getting shocked. Every time the rat gets shocked, it presses the lever, and the next shock is delayed for several minutes. If that lever is then made nonoperational, so it has no effect on the timing of the next shock, the rats still have a lower occurrence of stress-related diseases (such as ulcers and infections) because they *think* they still have control over the shocks. An interesting comparison can be made to people working under high-stress conditions, such as during a period of corporate layoffs. For many workers, this situation is one of high instability and low control (thus high stress), while for others, perhaps those in a department that will be unaffected by job cuts, there is much less stress (and fewer health problems).

This last part, about control, does *not* mean that you need to try to gain a high degree of control over every aspect of your life—because trying to do so can actually *increase* your cortisol levels. Instead, for most of us, it means doing your best, as the saying goes, to control those things you can control and to accept those things you cannot change (or have no control over).

As mentioned earlier, even though the first aspect of the SENSE program deals with managing and avoiding stressful situations, it is not the focus of this book to emphasize the many stress-management techniques that are available (see Resources for some recommendations). Despite the proven fact that the stress-management/stress-avoidance approach can be very helpful for some people, for others the very idea of incorporating relaxation techniques into their already hectic lives simply adds another source of stress (not good). For those folks, *The Cortisol Connection* offers what may be a more realistic set of cortisol-control recommendations: A plan that emphasizes sleep (one of the most effective ways to "manage" cortisol), exercise, nutrition, and supplements. The last SENSE recommendation—evaluation—reminds us that stress levels fluctuate and change, so our approach to controlling stress needs to be flexible enough to change with these fluctuating patterns (more about this in Chapter 12).

GET SOME SLEEP!

If you're like most people, you understand that stress management can be used effectively to help you deal with stressful events. After reading the previous chapters, you now know that effectively managing your stress response will help you maintain your cortisol levels within a more normal range. What you may *not* know, however, is that as little as a night or two of good, sound, restful sleep may do more for controlling your cortisol levels and reducing your long-term risk for many chronic diseases than a whole lifetime of stress-management classes. Here's why.

When you were just a few months old, a mere babe, your brain had you programmed to sleep about eighteen hours a day—not a very stressful existence. Upon reaching adulthood—say about twenty years of age—your nightly allotment of sleep had been slashed to less than seven hours (six hours and fifty-four minutes, according to the National Sleep Foundation). That's around two hours less than the eight to nine hours recommended by sleep experts for optimal physical and mental health. Progressive changes in your brain's internal clock (the suprachiasmatic nucleus), combined with alterations in your patterns of hormone secretion, have you going to bed later and waking up earlier with each successive decade, resulting in nearly thirty minutes less sleep per night with each passing decade. By the time we reach our thirties and forties, we're getting 80 percent less time in the most restful "slow-wave" period of sleep (as compared to our teenage years), and by the time we hit our fifties and sixties, we get almost no uninterrupted deep sleep. (We still get *some* deep sleep, but it tends to come in short fragments that do little in terms of recovery and repair for mind and body.)

What does this lack of sleep mean for your cortisol levels? It means that the average fifty-year-old has nighttime cortisol levels more than twelve times higher than the average thirty-year-old—yikes! Perhaps the worst piece of news is that not only will an inadequate quality or quantity of sleep result in elevated cortisol levels, but high cortisol will also limit both your ability to fall asleep and the amount of time that your mind spends in the most restful stages of deep sleep. This sets you up for a vicious cycle of poor sleep, elevated cortisol, and subtle changes in metabolism that leads you down the path toward chronic diseases. So get some sleep! A few suggestions for enhancing sleep are outlined in Chapter 12.

EXERCISE

Being active can help reduce some of the detrimental effects of chronic cortisol exposure. Exercise leads to production of dopamine and serotonin, both of which are "feel-good" anti-anxiety and antidepression chemicals produced in the brain and responsible for the well-known effect of "runner's high" that can help control the stress response. Researchers at Duke University have shown that exercise (thirty minutes per day, three to four days a week, for four months) can be as effective as prescription antidepressants in relieving symptoms of anxiety and depression.

Researchers at the University of Colorado have conducted several studies showing how exercise can reduce many of the detrimental effects of chronic stress. Regular participation in *moderate* exercise can reduce body fat, build muscle and bone, improve mental and emotional function, stimulate the immune response, and reduce appetite. The Colorado researchers have also shown that *extremes* of exercise, such as that undertaken by overtrained endurance athletes, can reverse these benefits by elevating cortisol levels, increasing body fat, interfering with mental and emotional functioning, suppressing immune functioning, and increasing the risk of injury. Scientists at the National Institutes of Health have noted that regular exercise can also help patients with extremely elevated cortisol levels (those with a condition known as Cushing's syndrome) prevent many of the metabolic derangements and much of the tissue destruction normally seen during the course of the disease.

> *Josh,* a real estate agent, husband, and father of four, was a perfect candidate for developing many of the adverse health conditions associated with stress and elevated cortisol levels. Despite knowing that exercise would be a great outlet for his stress, Josh felt that his irregular work schedule (long hours, nights, and weekends) meant that he had no time for a regular exercise program. However, by treating his daily exercise as a "client" and actually scheduling that time into his agenda, he was finally able to begin adhering to a regular program of jogging and lifting weights three times per week. Through exercise, Josh was able to harness his body's own fight-or-flight hormonal system to help reduce stress and balance his cortisol levels. The results for Josh have been most noticeable in terms of his energy levels and degree of creativity—both of which have impacted favorably on his real estate brokerage and his family life.

Good for Josh for managing to wedge a regular exercise regimen into his weekly schedule. But what about you? You may have joined gyms, tried jogging, and spent big bucks on fancy treadmills and stationary cycles that now serve mostly as coatracks—yet nothing seems to stick. Hints for alternate ways to work some physical activity into your normal daily routine are included in Chapter 12. (Additionally, check out the Resources section for books on the topic of exercise.)

NUTRITION

Eating right is also an important part of counteracting the effects of cortisol (big surprise). Proper diet can help modulate inflammatory responses in the body, while also promoting tissue repair. When it comes to "proper" diet, however, things can get a bit complicated. Many excellent books have been written on the topic of optimizing diet (see the Resources section). Instead of rehashing those nutritional recommendations, the following general suggestions are presented to help you craft your own cortisol-controlling diet plan.

What to Avoid?

One of the most positive antistress decisions you can make in terms of your diet is to cut down your use of alcohol, caffeine, and dietary supplements containing stimulants (such as ephedra). Does this mean you have to swear off any enjoyment of cola, coffee, tea, chocolate, wine, or beer? Certainly not, but it is important to understand that too much caffeine or related stimulants can send the already-stimulated nervous system from a state of heightened alertness into a state of nervousness and anxiety. In other people, alcohol can bear the same series of effects. Despite the fact that many people reach for a drink to calm their nerves (which it can do quite nicely), alcohol also acts as a diuretic to make the body lose water. This diuretic action often leaves a person in a dehydrated state, which the body perceives as a stressor, resulting in— you guessed it—elevated cortisol levels. Furthermore, alcohol can increase the occurrence of nighttime awakenings, an effect that is likely to counteract the otherwise restorative effects of sleep.

Dietary supplements targeted to weight loss and weight maintenance represent the largest category in the entire supplement industry. The key problem, however, is that many of the most popular dietary supplements on the market can actually increase cortisol levels in the body and make long-term weight control more difficult—primarily because they deliver an excessive dose of stimulants. Even though many of these supplements can be quite effective in suppressing appetite and increasing energy expenditure over a few short weeks (plenty of studies show this to be true), when used at high doses they also cause stress at the tissue and cellular levels. The body perceives this stimulant-mediated stress in the very same way that it perceives other forms of stress, and it responds by increasing the body's secretion of cortisol, which effectively sabotages any weight-loss successes experienced in the first few weeks of use. Taking supplements of this type can certainly help you lose weight, but when taken to excess they actually hurt your chances of long-term weight maintenance because of this effect of increasing cortisol levels.

Among the most important supplements to avoid at high doses are the herbal stimulants such as ma huang (ephedra), *Sida cordifolia* (ephedra), guarana (caffeine), *Citrus aurantium* (synephrine), coleus (forskolin), and yohimbe (yohimbine)—all of which increase the output of adrenaline and cortisol from the adrenal glands (and all of which are covered in more detail in the next chapter).

What to Eat?

We have the "what to avoid" part out of the way; now for the more interesting part about what to eat. When it comes to designing an antistress diet, the most important consideration is to maintain a balanced intake of the major macronutrients (protein, carbohydrates, and fats) along with the micronutrients (vitamins, minerals, and phytonutrients; see Chapter 7 for a detailed discussion of the role played by vitamins and minerals in combating the effects of stress and cortisol).

By selecting your blend of *macronutrients* from among the "right" kinds of foods—brightly colored fruits and veggies teamed with whole grains and lean cuts of meat, poultry, and fish—the vast majority of your *micronutrient* needs will automatically be satisfied. For example, a balanced breakfast of a scrambled egg, a piece of whole-grain toast, and a glass of orange juice provides a powerful dose of antistress nutrients. It contains protein (in the egg), carbohydrates (in the toast and juice), B vitamins (in the toast), antioxidants (in the juice), and phytonutrients (carotenoid lutein in the egg, citrus bioflavonoids in the juice, and lignans in the toast).

Phytonutrients are specialized vitaminlike compounds found in plants (*phyto-* means *plant*) that provide numerous health benefits. In general, the brighter in color the fruit or vegetable, the higher the content of particular phytonutrients. For example, lycopene, a red carotenoid, is found at high levels in tomatoes, while another carotenoid, beta-carotene, is responsible for the orange color of carrots and sweet potatoes. A simple (and fun) way to maximize your intake of phytonutrients and other micronutrients is to "color" your diet by trying to eat as many different colored fruits and vegetables as possible. Try shooting for five different colors each day: one serving each that is red (tomato), blue or purple (berries), yellow (melon), orange (carrot), and green (broccoli)—or whatever colors you can find. (Note: French fries do not count as a yellow vegetable.)

In terms of the macronutrients, many dieticians and nutritionists forget the concept of balance by guiding their clients toward a diet high in complex carbohydrates. While it is perfectly acceptable for most of us to focus our diet on increasing the amount of complex carbohydrates we eat, we must not forget to balance those carbohydrates with proper amounts of protein, fat, and fiber. During anxious or highly stressful times, we may even crave carbohydrates such as bread and sweets. Part of this is due to the effect of cortisol to suppress insulin function, increase blood-sugar levels, and stimulate appetite. In addition, however, your brain may urge you to eat more carbohydrates because they can act as a "tranquilizer" of sorts by increasing brain levels of serotonin (the neurotransmitter that calms us down). Unfortunately, while caving into the urges and chowing down on the carbs may give you a euphoric feeling for a few minutes, you'll surely pay for it later in the form of low energy levels, mood swings, more cravings, and a tendency toward weight gain.

Then there's the opposite problem. Some popular dietary advice takes the view that proteins are "good" and carbohydrates are "bad." Following such misguided instruction leads people to consume too much protein and not enough carbohydrate, again missing the point that what they should be striving for is the right balance of each. Achieving the right balance is of key importance, because each of the macronutrients performs a different primary role in the body. Protein can be thought of as the primary tissue builder (and rebuilder) because it helps us to maintain lean muscle mass. On the other hand, consuming more protein than a person needs, as one might do when using some of the very high protein bodybuilding drink mixes, can lead to dehydration and bloating. Carbohydrate consumption is vital because it serves as the primary fuel for the brain (which cannot use any other fuel source as efficiently) as well as a metabolic enhancer to encourage the body to use fat as a fuel source. A popular saying among metabolic physiologists is "fat burns in the flame of carbohydrate," which means that the breakdown products of carbohydrate metabolism are required for the optimal breakdown of stored body fat and the conversion of that fat into energy. Finally, both fat and fiber are needed to round out the balanced macronutrient mix because they both work to slow digestion and absorption of carbohydrates, control blood-sugar levels, and induce satiety (feelings of fullness). Additionally, certain kinds of dietary fat provide our only sources of the essential fatty acids (EFAs), linoleic acid and linolenic acid. These have been shown to help lower cholesterol and blood pressure, reduce the risk of heart disease, stroke, and possibly some kinds of cancer, and prevent dry hair and skin.

Protein Needs

That's all well and good: We need to have *some* carbohydrate and *some* protein at every meal—but how much? Let's start with our protein requirements. Very good research over the past decade or so shows that people who do a moderate amount of regular exercise (which you should be doing anyway for its cortisol-control benefits) need between 1.2 and 1.8 grams of protein per kilogram of body weight per day. You don't need to worry about all the mathematical gibberish, but you do need to understand that this means that a smaller person will need less protein in a given day than a larger person, simply because the larger person has more mass to support. For a 140-pound person, the math works out to about 77–115 grams of protein per day (let's say the average is 100 grams). For a 200-pound person, the protein requirement works out to 110–165 grams per day (we'll average that to 140 grams). Now, assuming that you're eating five to six small meals/snacks per day (as you should for optimal energy levels, appetite control, and fat metabolism), this amount of protein breaks down to about 20 grams per meal for the 140-pound person and not quite 30 grams per meal for the 200-pound person. Remember that eating more protein than this at each meal will not do anything extra in terms of muscle building; it will just add calories to your diet and increase your risk of becoming dehydrated and having gas.

Carbohydrate Needs

The next piece of the puzzle—how much carbohydrate you need—is determined largely by your weight-loss needs and your exercise patterns. If you need to lose weight, then you'll want to stay toward the low end of the recommended range (but avoid going too much lower, because fat metabolism will suffer). If you find yourself doing more than 30 minutes of exercise each day, then you'll want to be toward the high end of the recommended range (but not too much above it because of problems with insulin, blood-sugar control, and weight gain). So how much? First of all, let's realize that your brain wants to use carbohydrates (and carbohydrates only) for its energy needs. This amount generally works out to be about 100 grams of carbohydrate per day; without that amount, brain function slows down, you feel less "sharp," and your ability to concentrate is compromised. That said, you need at least 100 grams of carbohydrate (balanced with protein) in your daily diet. Do you need more? If you are also exercising (which you should be), then you'll need another 200–250 grams to support the needs of your muscles during intense efforts. Keeping in mind that "fat burns in the flame of carbohydrate," and that you should be eating five to six meals/snacks per day, then the math works out to be about 50–60 grams of carbohydrate per meal.

Putting all of the above mumbo jumbo together will have you consuming five to six meals/snacks per day, each composed of 20–30 grams of protein plus 50–60 grams of carbohydrate, which works out to a total caloric level of 280–360 calories per meal. Add to each meal/snack 3–5 grams of fiber (which contains no calories) and 3–5 grams of fat (30–40 additional calories) and you get optimal blood-sugar control, appetite regulation, enhanced fat metabolism, increased energy levels, better mood, and many more benefits.

Also check out the "Nutrition" section in Chapter 12, which provides tools for gauging appropriate serving sizes to meet these requirements. And if you want even more specific guidance, take a look at the Appendix, which contains several daily food plans for different calorie levels, plus tips for calculating your daily caloric needs.

Becky, like millions of people, was constantly fighting a losing battle against her weight and her hunger—especially in the late afternoon and early evening when she was most likely to crave a sweet snack. When her stress went up, so did her eating and her body weight. Unfortunately, as much as she was committed to doing what she thought to be the "right" things for weight loss, by skipping breakfast and following an extremely low-fat diet for the rest of the day she was using the wrong weapons in her battle of the bulge.

Becky's solution was to completely revamp her dietary regimen so that she ate something every three to four hours
throughout the day. That "something"—whether a meal or a
snack—was balanced to provide moderate amounts of carbohydrate and protein to help control blood sugar and regulate
appetite. The immediate benefits for Becky were a dramatic
decrease in her afternoon and evening cravings, an easier time
sticking to her diet, and a ten-pound loss of body fat within two
months.

SUPPLEMENTS

With all this emphasis on getting enough sleep, doing some exercise, and eating the right amounts of macronutrients and
micronutrients, where do dietary supplements fit in? Aside from
avoiding the several herbal stimulants mentioned above (which
can *increase* cortisol levels), a variety of dietary supplements exist
that can help to control the hypersecretion of cortisol, keeping it
within normal ranges even when a person is under stress.

Whether one's exposure to stress is the result of physical or
psychological factors, the response mounted by the body's hormonal system is exactly the same (and just as detrimental). This
means physical stressors such as suboptimal nutrition (dieting),
extremes of exercise, or inadequate sleep will affect the body in
many of the same ways as psychological stressors such as concerns
about body image, worry, and anger. No matter what source of
stress a person is exposed to, the body proceeds through a systemic
stress response that increases levels of cortisol and leads to many
of the associated declines in health. However, advances in nutritional science have shown that a wide variety of dietary and
herbal ingredients can instead assist the body in mounting an
adaptive response to stress and help to minimize or control some of
these systemic effects of stress. These natural products represent a
logical and convenient approach for many people who are subjected to stressors on a daily basis, for example from work,
finances, and/or the environment. For most of us most of the time,

removing the stressor (avoiding it) is an impossible option, no matter how desirable that option may be. Think about it: We all have to work (stress!), we all have to pay our bills on time (stress!), many of us have to sit in rush-hour traffic (stress!), and we all have family and interpersonal relationships that don't always go smoothly (stress!). Most of us also know that we *should* be eating better and that we *should* be getting more exercise (both of which can help control the stress response)—but the reality of our busy lives means that other things often take priority over exercise (job, kids, spouse, chores, you name it). In addition, the very concept of taking time out of those busy schedules for a yoga or meditation class is downright laughable, even though we know it would likely do us a lot of good.

For many, the only logical solution to managing an overactive stress response may be the use of certain dietary supplements to help control the body's excessive exposure to cortisol. These high-stress/high-cortisol episodes typically occur before bed, first thing in the morning, following meals, and during times that we all recognize as stressful (traffic jams, work deadlines, etc.). By keeping cortisol levels within a normal range, many of the adverse effects of acute and chronic stress can be held at bay—and taking the right combination of dietary supplements can be a safe, effective, and convenient approach for doing so.

As of this writing, the most promising cortisol-control supplements include the following (each of these is covered in more detail in Chapters 6 through 11):

Vitamins and Minerals for Stress Adaptation

Daily use of these is recommended for everybody from Stressed Jess to Strained Jane to Relaxed Jack.

- B-complex vitamins

- vitamin C

- magnesium

Supplements for Targeted Cortisol Control

Daily use is recommended for Stressed Jess and Strained Jane, but Relaxed Jack needs these supplements only during periods of especially high stress.

- magnolia bark

- epimedium

- theanine

- phytosterols

- phosphatidylserine

Support Supplements for Use During Heightened Stress

Occasional use only is recommended for Stressed Jess and Strained Jane when they need additional help relaxing or sleeping. Relaxed Jack generally has no additional need for supplements beyond those for targeted cortisol control.

- ashwagandha

- ginseng

- schisandra

- rhodiola

- kava kava

- valerian

- St. John's wort

- 5-HTP

- SAM-e

The next several chapters focus on helping you personalize a supplement program for your own specific needs. But first, how does one go about choosing and using dietary supplements? Where should you shop for supplements, and how do you select the best brand? Should you use supplements if you're taking prescription medications? Can supplements make up for an inadequate diet?

These are all good questions, and the following section answers them—and more.

GUIDELINES FOR CHOOSING AND USING DIETARY SUPPLEMENTS

Without a doubt, dietary supplements have widespread usage and appeal—to the tune of almost $17 billion in annual sales in the United States alone. Approximately 85 percent of Americans have used dietary supplements at one time or another, and more than 60 percent of the population are regular users of supplements (using them on most days of the week).

Despite the large number of people currently buying and using dietary supplements, however, a huge gap often exists between the practice of supplementation and the knowledge behind those choices and usage patterns. For example, while virtually 100 percent of adults consult their doctors or pharmacists about how to use prescriptions, less than half discuss dietary supplements with a health-care professional. In addition, many consumers are not careful about recommended dosages for supplements—and the common assumption that "if one is good, more is better" can pose serious health consequences for some supplement users.

It is very important that you discuss your use of dietary supplements with your health-care provider. In many cases that health professional will not be an expert in nutrition or supplementation, but the knowledge that you are supplementing your diet will at least alert them to issues such as the possibility for drug interactions or blood thinning.

It is also important that supplements be used responsibly. Just because they're not prescription drugs, it is dangerous to think that they can be used indiscriminately. Chapters 6 through 11 of this book can be used as a sort of handbook for supplements that target cortisol control, and the case studies presented throughout the book can help you decide on the most appropriate use of these supplements for your particular situation. For supplement recommendations in areas other than cortisol control, a consultation with a qualified nutritionist, dietician, herbalist, or nutritionally oriented physician is appropriate. Rather than blindly picking one of these consultants out of the yellow pages, you can check with the following organizations to find a qualified supplement consultant in your area:

American Nutraceutical Association (www.americanutra.com)
American College of Nutrition (www.am-coll-nutr.org)
American Dietetic Association (www.eatright.org)
SupplementWatch, Inc. (www.supplementwatch.com)

However, for some of the more straightforward supplement questions and answers, the following information can help guide you in choosing and using the right supplements in the proper manner.

CHOOSING SUPPLEMENTS

Below, I've answered some of the most common questions about how to choose among the many supplements available.

Q: Are natural forms of vitamins better than synthetic forms?

A: In most cases, natural and synthetic vitamins and minerals are handled by the body in exactly the same way. A good example of this is the B-complex vitamins, which can be obtained in supplements as "natural" B vitamins (usually from brewer's yeast or a similar substance) or as purified chemicals and listed on the product label as thiamin (B-1), riboflavin (B-2), niacin (B-3), and so forth. When either of these supplemental sources of B vitamins is consumed, the vitamins are absorbed, transported, and utilized by the body in exactly the same way—so we can say with confidence that there is no difference between natural and synthetic when it comes to B vitamins. Two interesting exceptions to this example are folic acid, which is better absorbed as the synthetic form (compared to natural forms found in foods), and vitamin E, which is far superior as the natural versus the synthetic form. In the case of vitamin E, very good scientific data exist showing that natural vitamin E is absorbed and retained in the body two to three times better than the synthetic forms. Natural vitamin E also costs a bit more than the synthetic variety, but the small added cost is more than justified by the higher activity.

Q: Should I choose a brand-name or generic vitamin/mineral supplement?

A: The ultimate answer to this question is less about generics or brand-name products than it is about choosing between supplements that provide "basic" versus "optimal" levels of particular nutrients. Therefore, your answer to this question will depend on two primary factors: How much money can you afford to spend on a supplement, and are you looking for a basic or an optimal supplement?

Many of the generic or private-label store-brand supplements on the market will do a satisfactory job of helping you meet the basic RDA (recommended daily allowance) levels for essential vitamins and minerals. The primary limitation with these generic products, and even with many brand-name supplements, is that the basic RDA levels of most vitamins and minerals fall far below the levels associated with optimal health and certainly below those needed for optimal cortisol control. Chapter 7 outlines many of the details surrounding the use of vitamins and minerals for cortisol control, but a couple of the most important are worth highlighting here:

With respect to the B vitamins, there is very good scientific evidence to support daily intakes at 200–500 percent of RDA levels for optimal stress response and cortisol control. These levels are two to five times higher than the levels found in most multivitamin products.

Calcium and magnesium are two minerals that are known to help regulate the body's stress response, yet most generic supplements and "one-tablet-a-day" type brand-name supplements provide only a small fraction of the 250–500 milligrams (mg) of calcium and the 125–250 mg of magnesium needed to aid cortisol control. The primary reason for skimping on the calcium and magnesium in these products is due not to costs (both are very cheap), but to space considerations in the capsules and tablets. Both calcium and magnesium are bulky minerals—that is, they take up a lot of space—so an optimal daily dosage requires more than a single capsule each day (and sometimes as many as four capsules depending on the mineral source).

The bottom line here is that everybody should take at least a basic multivitamin/multimineral supplement—and virtually any product, generic or brand-name, on the shelf at Wal-Mart, Rite-Aid, or your local grocery store will satisfy the basic RDA-level requirements. However, if you are interested in a supplement that delivers more than the rock-bottom levels of cortisol-controlling nutrients, and if you can afford to spend a little more on your daily supplement regimen, then you will want to consider a multivitamin/mineral supplement that provides higher levels of B-complex vitamins, calcium, and magnesium.

Q: What should I consider when I am shopping for herbal supplements?

A: When it comes to selecting herbal supplements, the situation can quickly get very confusing. Because herbals are really a form of natural medicine, it is crucial that you select the right form of the herb so that you get the safest and most effective product. Herbal supplements are absolutely an area in which generic products are *not* equivalent to brand-name products. It is vitally important to select either the exact product that has been used in clinical studies, or a product that contains a chemically equivalent form of the herb that has been studied. The easiest way for most consumers to select a safe and effective herb is to select only those extracts that have been "standardized" to provide a uniform level of the key active ingredients in each batch of the product (see the supplement descriptions in Chapters 6 through 11 for details on these standards). The best scenario would be to select only those specific *products* that have undergone clinical studies of their own (rather than selecting products that contain *ingredients* on which studies have been conducted)—but there are far fewer finished products that have been subjected to clinical testing than there are raw ingredients (echinacea, St. John's wort, etc.) that have been evaluated in such research.

Q: Where is the best place to buy supplements?

A: The preceding three questions should offer enough general guidance to help you weed through the many less desirable supplement products on the market and select products that can make a difference in your overall health. With the explosive growth in the supplement market over the past decade, consumers can now find vitamins, minerals, herbs, and other supplements for sale in a variety of places— including specialty supplement stores, natural-foods stores, drugstores, grocery stores, discount department stores, and through direct marketing, infomercials, catalog sales, and the Internet. Is any of these outlets better than the others? Not really—but they each have their own particular niche.

For example, the least expensive "bargain" products will be found at supermarkets and discount department stores (e.g., Wal-Mart), but these products may suffer from many of the problems outlined above with regard to basic versus optimal supplementation. Supplements that are a step above the cheapest and most basic of products can typically be found at drugstores, natural-foods markets, and specialty supplement outlets. These are the middle-of-the-road products that do a decent job of balancing high-quality and optimal nutrient levels with moderate prices.

The most expensive products, and those with the widest range in terms of quality, safety, and effectiveness, are typically sold through direct sales channels such as the Internet, catalogs, and independent sales agents. In some cases, these products are designed to deliver optimal levels of all nutrients in the most bioavailable forms, but the obvious downside is their high price. In other cases, all you get is the high price—without any of the optimal levels of the crucial nutrients. So how can you differentiate between these premium-priced products? By asking to see the results from their clinical studies. Products in this "premium" category will almost certainly need to justify their high price with strong scientific evidence to support their claims and to show that their product is justified at this price. If the company cannot provide you with scientific evidence to support its premium products, then you are well advised to look elsewhere for your supplement.

USING SUPPLEMENTS

After you have selected your supplements with the help of the above information, the following guidelines can help you to use those supplements in the proper manner (that is, so you optimize both safety and effectiveness):

- Remember that a dietary supplement is just that—meaning that it is meant to be added to an otherwise healthy diet. It is not meant to substitute for a balanced diet or to make up for a poor diet.

- Follow the dosage recommendations on the package. The recommended dosage is important for safety and effectiveness—especially for herbals and other supplements that combine multiple ingredients. Don't make the mistaken assumption that if one tablet is recommended per day, two or three will be even better.

- Keep all dietary supplements in a safe place—away from heat and light that may accelerate their breakdown, and away from children who may accidentally ingest them.

- Talk to your health-care provider about any dietary supplements you are taking. If you are on any form of prescription or over-the-counter medication, talk with your doctor or pharmacist *before* using *any* supplements.

CHAPTER 6

Dietary Supplements to Avoid

As indicated in Chapter 4, high cortisol levels are associated with being overweight, and yet at the same time cortisol levels are elevated by dieting and by cognitive dietary restraint (a fancy term for thinking about dieting). It is no wonder, then, that people who are under chronic or repeated stress tend to struggle with their weight, their appetite, and their energy levels—all of which are impacted by the elevated cortisol levels associated with their stress. It would seem to be a virtual miracle for a dietary supplement to come along with claims of increasing weight loss, suppressing appetite, and boosting energy levels. In fact, this supplement would almost seem to be tailor-made for people under stress, because it addresses three of the key factors that lead them down the path to weight gain.

The "miracle" supplements described above fall into a category of herbal stimulants that function as *sympathomimetics*—meaning they mimic some of the effects of the body's own sympathetic (stimulant) hormones such as epinephrine and norepinephrine, either by increasing the secretion of those hormones or by reducing their breakdown. Among the most popular herbals in this category are *Ephedra sinensis* (ma huang), *Citrus aurantium* (synephrine),

Coleus forskohlii (forskolin), *Paullinia cupana* (guarana/caffeine), and *Pausinystalia yohimbe* (yohimbine)—but many other plant species contain related stimulant compounds. Each of these herbs acts as a general stimulant on many parts of the body simultaneously, including the lungs (where they can open bronchioles to make breathing easier), the heart and blood vessels (where they increase heart rate and constrict arteries to increase blood pressure), and even the adrenal glands (where they stimulate the secretion of epinephrine and cortisol). Because of these wide-ranging actions in many tissues, the herbal stimulants are also frequently associated with a number of adverse side effects such as headaches, insomnia, elevated blood pressure, irritability, and heart palpitations. But perhaps the side effect that provokes the most concern is the large increase in cortisol levels caused by these substances.

The widespread popularity of the herbal stimulants—most notably ephedra—is due largely to the fact that they work. Ephedra and related supplements are well known to kill appetite and increase energy levels, so you either exercise more or you fidget more, but either way, you burn some extra calories. This means that over the course of a month or two, the herbal stimulant products will help a person drop a few more pounds than he otherwise would have been able to do on his own. The downside, however, is the fact that while the short-term effects of these compounds are beneficial for weight loss (by reducing appetite and increasing caloric expenditure), the longer-term increase in cortisol levels is detrimental for weight-loss efforts. Why? Because, as outlined in Chapter 4, that increase in cortisol levels will increase hunger, slow fat metabolism, eat away at muscles and bones, sap energy, wreck mood, and generally thwart attempts to maintain a healthy body weight.

So here we have a class of weight-loss supplements that provides some actual benefits when used for a few weeks, but then turns on the user to cause a series of metabolic changes in the body that *promote* weight gain over several months. If that news isn't already bad enough, it also appears that the tendency of ephedra and related compounds to cause weight gain over a longer period of time is even stronger when the user is experiencing an additional stressor (and dieting is a stressor). Researchers from Lausanne University in Switzerland found that as little as two days of ephedra consumption, at 40 milligrams (mg) per day, reduced glucose uptake and oxidation by 25 percent. When subjects were under additional stress, the fall in glucose uptake and oxidation exceeded 50 percent! This means ephedra supplements inhibit the body's ability to use glucose as an energy source, so blood-sugar levels climb, fat metabolism shuts off, and hunger comes raging back. Similar findings have been noted for forskolin (the active ingredient in *Coleus forskohlii*), yohimbine (the active ingredient in *Pausinystalia yohimbe*), and caffeine (the active ingredient in *Paullinia cupana*, also known as guarana). For example, around 200 mg of caffeine (about the amount contained in two cups of coffee and in a single dose of many weight-loss supplements) will increase blood levels of cortisol by 30 percent within one hour.

What we see in the longer-term studies of herbal stimulants is a persistent elevation in plasma cortisol levels caused by a stresslike neuroendocrine response to stimulation of the brain and the adrenal glands. In animal studies, this type of nervous-system stimulation leads not only to elevated cortisol levels, but also to reductions in levels of growth hormone and thyroid stimulating hormone, both of which are involved in keeping us lean.

So what to do? The most prudent approach would be to completely avoid these herbal stimulants in favor of a more balanced approach to promoting weight loss, such as eating several small meals spaced throughout the day, getting a balanced intake of protein/carbs/fat/fiber, and taking regular aerobic exercise plus resistance training. That said, millions of people are likely to keep using products that have herbal stimulants in them. Despite the long-term risk to overall health and the sabotage such supplements can bring to a person's weight-maintenance efforts, the quick-fix promise of dropping a few extra pounds in a few weeks is simply too much for many people to resist. If you *do* decide to use any of these herbal stimulants, please do so with extreme caution—and try to curb your use of them after one month. At the very least, the cortisol-*raising* effects of the herbal stimulants should be counteracted by combining their use with one of the cortisol-lowering herbs outlined in Chapter 8. It is unlikely that the cortisol-controlling supplements will counteract either the appetite-control or the thermogenic/fat-burning effects of the herbal stimulants, but they will certainly lessen the adverse side effects of elevated cortisol.

The rest of the chapter provides brief summaries of each of the most popular herbal stimulants used in weight-loss supplements.

MA HUANG/EPHEDRA

Ma huang is a Chinese herb that is also referred to as *Chinese ephedra (Ephedra sinensis)* and *herbal ephedrine*. The active compounds—ephedra or ephedrine alkaloids—are also found in other herbals such as Mormon tea and *Sida cordifolia*, and may be referred to by common names such as desert tea, Mexican tea, sea grape, and many others. Overall, about forty species of plants contain versions of ephedra.

Ma huang and its various herbal cousins function as sympathomimetics, the effects of which are described earlier in this chapter. Ephedrine is considered a *nonselective sympathomimetic*, which means that it acts as a general stimulant on many parts of the body simultaneously (lungs, heart, blood vessels, adrenal glands, and others). Therefore, it can give users a boost or pickup similar to what they might feel after a cup or two of strong coffee. By mimicking the effects of epinephrine, ephedra can increase the output of blood from the heart, enhance muscle contractility, raise blood-sugar levels, and open bronchial pathways for easier breathing. In many cases, ephedra can result in a temporary suppression of appetite, which may help efforts aimed at dietary restriction and weight loss.

The research findings concerning the effects of ma huang and other ephedra-containing products are equivocal; some studies show absolutely no beneficial effect, some studies show a modest increase in weight loss, and still other studies suffer from high numbers of subjects dropping out due to unpleasant side effects. Because ephedrine is a stimulant, it is logical that either a single dose or chronic repeated use would elevate metabolic rate somewhat (meaning the user would burn more calories at rest and during exercise). Various studies of overweight men and women have shown that the combination of ephedrine (20–40 mg) and caffeine (200–400 mg) produces a slight increase in resting metabolism.

The Food and Drug Administration (FDA) has received more than a thousand reports of adverse side effects from consumers using supplements containing ephedrine alkaloids. Complaints have ranged from nervous-system and cardiovascular-system effects such as elevated blood pressure and heart palpitations, to insomnia, irritability, headaches, and serious adverse effects such as seizures, stroke, heart attack, and even death (about fifteen to twenty thus far). Most of these adverse events occurred in otherwise healthy, young to middle-aged adults using the products for weight control or increased energy.

Health Warning for
Ephedra-Containing Dietary Supplements

Virtually all dietary supplements that contain ephedra alkaloids also carry a strong warning on their label. It reads something like the following:

Women who are pregnant or nursing should avoid using ephedra-containing products. Keep out of reach of children. Avoid using ephedrine-containing products if you have high blood pressure, heart or thyroid disease, diabetes, difficulty in urination due to prostate enlargement, or if taking monoamine oxidase (MAO) inhibitors or any other prescription drug. Reduce or discontinue use if nervousness, tremor, irritability, rapid heartbeat, sleeplessness, loss of appetite, or nausea occurs.

Across the range of studies that have been conducted on products containing ephedra for weight loss, the total amount of ephedrine ingested per day has ranged between 60 and 75 mg of ephedrine alone (usually in three doses of 20–25 mg each) or 20–40 mg of ephedrine combined with 200–400 mg of caffeine. It is important to note, however, that these dosage recommendations should be considered in light of recent studies showing that the levels of ephedra alkaloids can vary by as much as 1,000 percent from one dietary supplement to another.

The purified versions of ephedra (ephedrine and pseudoephedrine) found in many over-the-counter cold medicines have the very same effect on cortisol levels (raising them). However, in contrast to ephedra-based weight-loss supplements, which might be used for many weeks at a time (and thus lead to chronically high cortisol levels), typical cold remedies are used for no more than a few days in a row and thus would cause only a temporary rise in cortisol levels.

Should you decide to use ephedra-containing products, it is important to understand that while the *short-term* effects (suppressed appetite and slight increase in caloric expenditure) might give your weight-loss efforts a boost, the *longer-term* effects (chronically elevated cortisol levels) will almost certainly sabotage your ability to maintain that weight loss. Therefore, ephedra supplements should be used for no more than six to twelve weeks, and even then, for optimal effect, they should be balanced with supplements that help to control cortisol levels.

GUARANA

Guarana (*Paullinia cupana*) comes from the seeds of a Brazilian plant. Traditional uses of guarana by natives of the Amazonian rain forest include adding crushed seeds to foods and beverages for increasing alertness and reducing fatigue. As a dietary supplement, it's no wonder guarana is an effective energy booster; it contains about twice the caffeine found in coffee beans. Guarana seeds are about 3–4 percent caffeine, compared to the 1–2 percent in coffee beans. Concentrated guarana extracts, however, can contain as much as 40–50 percent caffeine, with popular supplements delivering 50–200 mg of caffeine per day, about the same amount found in one or two cups of strong coffee. Guarana is generally considered to be as safe for healthy people as caffeine. As with any caffeine-containing substance, guarana extracts can lead to insomnia, nervousness, anxiety, headaches, high blood pressure, and heart palpitations.

The theory behind how guarana works is relatively straightforward. The major active constituents are caffeine (sometimes called *guaranine* to make the user think it's different in some way) and similar alkaloids such as theobromine and theophylline, which are also found in coffee and tea. Each of these compounds has well-known effects as nervous-system stimulants. As such, they may also bear some effect on increasing metabolic rate, suppressing appetite, and enhancing both physical and mental performance.

Most of the scientific evidence on caffeine as a general stimulant and an aid to exercise performance shows convincingly that caffeine is effective. As a weight-loss aid, although high doses of caffeine may somewhat suppress appetite, on its own it does not seem to be a very effective supplement for increasing caloric expenditure (thermogenesis). However, when combined with other stimulant-type supplements, such as ma huang (ephedra), it appears that caffeine can extend the duration of ephedra's action in suppressing appetite and increasing caloric expenditure; it is unknown whether caffeine may also increase the risk of adverse side effects.

Brad wanted to lose twenty pounds before his twenty-year high school reunion—and he only had a little more than two months to do it. The amount of weight Brad wanted to lose, and the time frame in which he wanted to lose it, meant that he would need to achieve a weight loss of about two pounds per week—an aggressive, but still achievable, objective. To help him reach his target weight, in addition to his diet and exercise program Brad was interested in taking one of the popular thermogenic ephedra/caffeine supplements used for suppressing appetite and increasing energy levels. Because high doses of both ephedra and caffeine are known to elevate cortisol levels, Brad also chose to follow a cortisol-control regimen that included the supplements epimedium (300 mg per day) and phosphatidylserine (25 mg per day). See Chapter 8 for more about these two supplements.

As the reunion approached, Brad was happy to see his weight dropping closer and closer to his goal. But he was most excited to see the primary benefits of his ephedra/caffeine supplement (appetite suppression and elevated energy levels) continue at their full effect, instead of dropping off after he'd used them for longer than a few weeks, as many of his friends had experienced. By using epimedium and phosphatidylserine to counteract the ephedra/caffeine-induced rise in his cortisol levels, Brad was able to extend the weight-loss benefits of his thermogenic supplement until the day of his reunion—and then to show up in front of his former classmates in a new slim and trim form.

SYNEPHRINE

Synephrine is the main active compound found in the fruit of a plant called *Citrus aurantium*. The fruit is also known as *zhi shi* in traditional Chinese medicine, and as *green orange, sour orange,* and *bitter orange* in other parts of the world. Synephrine is chemically very similar to the ephedrine found in a number of weight-loss and energy supplements that contain ma huang. But synephrine differs from ephedrine in that synephrine is considered a *semi-selective sympathomimetic* (because it targets some tissues, such as fat, more than it targets others, such as the heart) versus a *non-selective sympathomimetic* (like ephedra, which targets many tissues equally and thus often causes side effects). For example, although some high-dose ephedra-containing supplements have been associated with certain cardiovascular side effects such as elevated blood pressure and heart palpitations, researchers at Mercer University in Atlanta have shown that *Citrus aurantium* extract has no effect on hemodynamics such as heart rate and blood pressure because it targets fat tissue rather than heart tissue.

Because synephrine is a mild stimulant, similar in some ways to caffeine and ephedrine, it is thought to have similar effects in terms of providing an energy boost, suppressing appetite, and increasing metabolic rate and caloric expenditure. In traditional Chinese medicine, zhi shi is used to help stimulate *qi* (pronounced *chee*, and defined as the body's vital energy or life force), but in order to maximize the metabolic benefits of these extracts, total synephrine intake should probably be kept to a range of 2–10 mg per day.

A recent study in dogs suggests that synephrine and octopamine found in *Citrus aurantium* extracts can increase metabolic rate in a specific type of fat tissue known as brown adipose tissue (BAT). This effect would be expected to increase fat loss in humans, except for one small detail: Adult humans don't have any brown adipose tissue to speak of. Despite this fact, this claim still stands as one of the most overhyped promises on the weight-loss scene. Until very recently, synephrine-containing supplements existed solely because there were some interesting theories on how they *might* work to increase metabolic rate and promote significant weight loss. At this writing, there are at least two clinical studies showing that synephrine-containing supplements help promote weight loss, and at least three clinical studies showing enhanced thermogenesis (calorie expenditure) from these supplements. There is a great deal of research currently underway into the weight-loss benefits of synephrine and supplements with related thermogenic effects, leading researchers in the Department of Physiology at Georgetown University to conclude that "*Citrus aurantium* may be the best thermogenic substitute for ephedra."

YOHIMBE

Yohimbe (*Pausinystalia yohimbe*) comes from the bark of an African tree; the active compound, yohimbine, can also be found in high amounts in the South American herb quebracho (*Aspidosperma quebracho-blanco*). It has traditionally been used as a stimulant and aphrodisiac in West Africa and South America. In

the United States, yohimbe and quebracho are most often promoted in dietary supplements for treating impotence, stimulating
male sexual performance (often marketed as "herbal Viagra"), and
enhancing athletic performance (as an alternative to anabolic
steroids). More recently, however, yohimbe and quebracho have
also been showing up in dietary supplements focused toward promoting fat loss and muscle gain at the same time.

A purified extract from yohimbe bark yields an alkaloid called
yohimbine that is similar in structure to caffeine and ephedra; it is
regulated as a prescription medication used for treating erectile
dysfunction in males. Yohimbine functions as a monoamine oxidase (MAO) inhibitor to increase levels of the neurotransmitter
norepinephrine, but it also acts as a stimulator of the central nervous system, where it interacts with specific receptors (alpha-2
adrenergic receptors) and may increase energy levels and promote
fat oxidation.

Although yohimbe is frequently promoted as a natural way to
increase testosterone levels for muscle building, strength enhancement, and fat loss, there is no solid scientific proof that yohimbe
is either anabolic or thermogenic. Results from a few small trials
show that purified synthetic yohimbine can increase blood flow to
the genitals, an effect that may occur in both men and women. As
such, yohimbe bark, which contains small amounts of natural
yohimbine, may be effective in alleviating some mild forms of both
"psychological" and "physical" impotence. In the few studies conducted on the purified form of yohimbine, only about 30 percent
of subjects reported beneficial effects in terms of erectile function
and sexual performance.

As the number of yohimbe products on the retail market
increases, concerns about their safety are raised because of the
reported toxicity of yohimbine, the plant's major alkaloid and
active ingredient. Reported side effects from yohimbe use include
minor complaints such as headaches, anxiety, and tension, as well
as more serious adverse events, including high blood pressure, elevated heart rate, heart palpitations, and hallucinations. People with
high blood pressure and kidney disease should avoid supplements

containing yohimbe, as should women who are, or who could become, pregnant (due to a potential risk of miscarriage). Also, caution should be used when taking yohimbe in combination with certain foods containing tyramine (such as red wine, liver, and cheese) as well as with nasal decongestants or diet aids containing ephedrine or phenylpropanolamine, which could lead to danger-ous blood-pressure fluctuations.

COLEUS

Coleus (*Coleus forskohlii*) is part of the mint family of plants and has long been used in India, Thailand, and parts of Southeast Asia as both a spice and an Ayurvedic medicine for treating heart ail-ments and stomach cramps. The roots of the plant are a natural source of forskolin, a compound that can increase cellular levels of cyclic adenosine monophosphate (cAMP), an effect that is theo-rized to influence many aspects of metabolism. The primary use of coleus extracts in modern dietary supplements is for a purported effect in promoting weight loss and stimulating muscle growth.

The theory behind *Coleus forskohlii* as a dietary supplement is that its content of forskolin can be used to stimulate adenylate cyclase activity, which will increase cAMP levels in the fat cell, which will in turn activate another enzyme (hormone-sensitive lipase) to start breaking down fat stores. The problem with this theory is that cAMP regulates the activity of hundreds of enzymes in each cell—and those enzymes can be quite different from cell to cell. For example, we know that in cell cultures (test-tube stud-ies), adding forskolin to fat cells will increase cAMP levels and stimulate lipolysis (breakdown of stored triglycerides into free fatty acids). Add that same forskolin to muscle cells, however, and the primary effect is to stimulate glycogenolysis (breakdown of stored glycogen into free glucose units). Add forskolin to liver cells and you get a stimulation of gluconeogenesis (synthesis of blood glucose from amino acid precursors).

Most of the work conducted on the actions of forskolin have been confined to test tubes, where researchers have been studying its actions in increasing cellular cAMP levels and the effects of cAMP on regulating various hormone/enzyme systems. There are no published trials showing that the supplement promotes either weight loss or increased lean body mass or any other health benefit in humans, though health food–industry publications frequently tout a small, poorly conducted trial of six overweight women in whom 500 mg of coleus extract per day for eight weeks caused a loss of body fat and an increase in muscle. These data are completely useless to us, as there was no blinding of subjects and no placebo control group, so there is no way to determine whether the weight loss was due to the supplement (which is highly unlikely) or to some other factor, such as a change in diet or exercise patterns (far more likely).

The typical dosage recommendations for coleus extracts are in the range of 100–300 mg per day (10–20 percent forskolin), which appears to be more than enough to induce a significant rise in blood levels of cortisol.

Summary

I hope the preceding information helps to put some of the "miracle" weight-loss claims for herbal stimulants into proper perspective. Far from being a stand-alone solution for weight maintenance, these supplements—while they offer the benefits of appetite control, enhanced energy levels, and increased caloric expenditure—absolutely must be used within the proper dosage range (and, even better, should be used in conjunction with at least one cortisol controller). At excessive doses, users risk adverse side effects, long-term elevations in cortisol levels, and the associated metabolic changes that can sabotage your weight-loss efforts.

But there is good news. The rest of this book profiles some of the supplements that are most effective for controlling stress, balancing cortisol levels, and dealing with many of the associated metabolic changes.

CHAPTER 7

Vitamins and Minerals for Stress Adaptation

It almost goes without saying that taking a general multivitamin and mineral supplement is a good idea for anybody who is under stress, maintains a hectic lifestyle, or needs more energy. Every energy-related reaction that takes place in the body relies in one way or another on vitamins and minerals as cofactors to make the reactions go. For example, B-complex vitamins are needed for metabolism of protein and carbohydrate; chromium is involved in carbohydrate handling; magnesium and calcium are needed for proper muscle contraction; zinc and copper are required as enzyme cofactors in nearly three hundred separate reactions; iron is needed to help shuttle oxygen in the blood—the list goes on and on.

It is fairly well accepted in the medical community that subclinical or marginal deficiencies of essential micronutrients, especially the B vitamins and magnesium, can lead to psychological and physiological symptoms that are related to stress. One study, published in 2000, looked at the effects of a multivitamin/mineral supplement on overall stress levels. The supplement was a water-soluble formula, composed of vitamins C (1,000 mg), B-1 (15 mg), B-2 (15 mg), B-3 (50 mg), B-6 (10 mg), B-12 (10 mcg), biotin (150 mcg), pantothenic acid (23 mg), calcium (100 mg), and magnesium (100 mg). For a period of thirty days, 150 volunteers who were prescreened for having high levels of stress consumed the supplement each morning with water, while another 150 "high-stress" volunteers received a placebo pill. Before and after the thirty-day supplementation period, researchers administered a battery of standardized stress tests. The test results showed a sta-tistically different and clinically important improvement in the overall stress index of the volunteers taking the multivitamin/ mineral supplement, but not in the placebo group. Another study (also a double-blind, placebo-controlled trial) of eighty healthy male volunteers found that twenty-eight days of treatment with a mineral supplement containing calcium, magnesium, and zinc sig-nificantly reduced anxiety and sensations of stress. These studies, and dozens like them, support the rationale behind using a general nutritional supplement as your antistress foundation on which to build a solid cortisol-control regimen.

"STRESS-FORMULA" MULTIVITAMINS

In an effort to capitalize on the huge market for "stress-reducing" products, many of the large pharmaceutical and dietary-supplement companies have introduced "stress-formula" multi-vitamin products. These formulations are based on available scien-tific evidence suggesting that certain nutrients may be needed at levels higher than the RDAs (recommended daily allowances) for optimal support of adrenal function and control of cortisol levels. For example, vitamin C supplementation at a dose of 1,000 mg per day improves the capacity of the adrenals to adapt to surgical stress by normalizing cortisol and ACTH in patients with lung cancer. Thiamin (vitamin B-1) is effective in reducing the typical increase in postsurgical secretion of cortisol from the adrenal glands. In one study, a combination of vitamins C, B-1, and B-6 was able to bring the pattern of cortisol secretion back into normal ranges following surgery. Pantothenic acid (vitamin B-5) is another required nutri-ent for proper functioning of the adrenal gland. Consumption of pantothenic acid by humans buffers the rise in cortisol during experimental stress, which suggests a potential benefit of vitamin B-5 in controlling the hypersecretion of cortisol during periods of stress. Overall, it makes little difference whether you decide to get your cortisol-controlling nutrients as part of a general multivitamin/ mineral product or from a more targeted "stress-tab" sort of formula; the important thing is that you *do* get them.

Without getting bogged down in too many details, we can outline some of the general ways in which essential nutrients (vitamins and minerals) help to counteract the detrimental health effects of chronic stress. For example, magnesium, a mineral that we most often think about in terms of both bone health and heart function, has been shown to reduce cortisol levels following exhaustive exercise in healthy male athletes. Zinc, a mineral that we commonly associate with both bone health and immune function, is known to alter adrenal metabolism when levels in the diet are either too high or too low. In one study, 25–50 mg of zinc (about two to three times the RDA) resulted in a significant fall in plasma cortisol levels in healthy volunteers (again, following an extreme exercise stress test that typically raises cortisol levels). Chromium, a mineral that we typically think of in terms of its benefits for blood-sugar control and appetite regulation, has been shown to help reduce serum cortisol in livestock (cattle and sheep) exposed to the stress of cross-country transport. In both groups of animals, those receiving chromium supplements also demonstrated a more robust immune-system function, as evidenced by fewer infections, compared to the animals receiving the placebo.

In addition to the observed effects of isolated nutrients on cortisol levels, there are numerous instances of general dietary alterations bearing a positive impact on reducing elevated cortisol levels. For example, one study of sodium restriction documented a drop in urinary levels of cortisol following one week on a sodium-restricted diet. Upon switching back to the higher-sodium diet, researchers observed a 30 percent increase in the body's production of cortisol within a few days. Dietary changes in protein and carbohydrate intake are also known to influence the body's handling of cortisol. In one study of athletes, consumption of an amino-acid solution (100 mg arginine, 80 mg ornithine, 70 mg leucine, 35 mg isoleucine, and 35 mg valine) resulted in a significant suppression of cortisol levels within sixty minutes. When it comes to carbohydrate consumption, numerous studies have demonstrated the cortisol-lowering benefits of carbohydrates, especially when they are consumed during exercise. In one notable study, after ten days on a high-carbohydrate diet, cortisol concentrations were significantly lower than after ten days on a lower-carbohydrate diet. Supplementing the diet with a carbohydrate-rich sports drink has also been shown to reduce serum cortisol during endurance exercise (compared to a placebo drink). High-fat diets, in contrast, have been shown in rodent studies to impair the body's ability to restore normal cortisol levels following stress.

So there you have it— cortisol metabolism, and indeed the entire underlying stress response, is influenced to a large degree by a person's intake of vitamins, minerals, and other nutrients. Knowing that to be true, a big step you can take in controlling your own stress response is to eat right and to take at least a basic multivitamin supplement (or even better, a comprehensive multivitamin/multimineral supplement). For more targeted cortisol-control activity, some nutrients appear to offer additional benefits; these are outlined in the sections that follow.

VITAMIN C

Vitamin C, also known as ascorbic acid, is a water-soluble vitamin needed by the body for hundreds of vital metabolic reactions. As a dietary supplement, vitamin C is consumed by more people than any other vitamin, mineral, or herbal product. Good food sources of vitamin C include all citrus fruits (oranges, grapefruit, lemons) as well as many other fruits and vegetables such as strawberries, tomatoes, broccoli, Brussels sprouts, peppers, and cantaloupe.

As a dietary supplement, vitamin C is generally regarded as a potent antioxidant and is generally consumed for the prevention of colds, stimulation of the immune system, promotion of wound healing, and to ward off some of the detrimental effects of stress (see also the discussion of vitamin C's immune-enhancing properties in Chapter 11). Because of the wide variety of reactions in which vitamin C plays a role, many claims are made about its value as a supplement. Perhaps the best-known function of vitamin C is as one of the key nutritional antioxidants, whereby it protects the body from free-radical damage. As a water-soluble vitamin, ascorbic acid performs its antioxidant functions within the aqueous portions of the blood and cells, and can help restore the antioxidant potential of vitamin E (a fat-soluble antioxidant).

As a preventive against infections such as influenza and other viruses, vitamin C is thought to strengthen cell membranes, thereby preventing entrance of the virus to the interior of the cell. Support of immune-cell function is another key role performed by vitamin C and one that may help fight infections in their early stages. The combined effects of cellular strengthening, collagen synthesis, and antioxidant protection are thought to account for the multifaceted approach by which vitamin C helps to counteract stress and maintain health.

In two separate studies about vitamin C supplementation (1,000–1,500 mg per day for one week), ultramarathon runners showed a 30 percent lower cortisol level in their blood when compared to runners receiving a placebo. In another study of healthy children undergoing treatment with synthetic corticosteroids, 1 gram (1,000 mg) of vitamin C, consumed three times a day for five days, resulted in significantly lower cortisol levels compared to healthy children given a placebo. In a study of lung-cancer patients, a dose of 2 grams of vitamin C, given daily for one week prior to surgery, was able to bring elevated cortisol levels (resulting from the surgery) back to normal ranges in a significantly shorter period of time compared to patients receiving a placebo.

It has been shown in numerous animal and human studies that even a subclinical deficiency of vitamin C (that is, a deficiency small enough not to produce results detectable by the usual clinical tests) will result in an elevation of plasma cortisol levels. In studies of various laboratory and livestock animals, even a marginal vitamin C deficiency produced a significant increase in plasma cortisol levels and an inhibition of immune function, both of which were reversed by adding vitamin C back into the diet. These suboptimal levels of vitamin C, and their resulting elevation in cortisol, may account at least in part for the immune-system suppression and mild depression observed in elderly volunteers. In one study, thirty elderly volunteers (ten women and twenty men) were given 1 gram of vitamin C daily for sixteen weeks. Results showed a significant decrease in serum cortisol in both groups, as well as a significant improvement in various parameters of immune function.

Vitamin C supplements are most often used as a way to prevent or reduce the symptoms associated with the common cold—and well over one hundred studies have been conducted in this area. In several of the largest studies, no effect on common-cold incidence was observed, indicating to many scientists that vitamin C has no preventive effects in normally nourished subjects who experience normal exposure to stress. However, a number of smaller, targeted studies, conducted in subjects under heavy acute physical stress, show that vitamin C decreases the incidence of the common cold by more than half. In other studies, healthy subjects consuming low levels of vitamin C (below 60 mg per day) experienced about one-third fewer colds following vitamin C supplementation.

In most cases, it appears that although the most important and dramatic preventive effects of vitamin C supplementation are experienced by individuals with low vitamin C intakes, those with an average daily consumption from foods may also benefit from supplemental levels—especially during periods of heightened stress. In support of an elevated vitamin C intake, an expert scientific panel recently recommended increasing the current RDA for vitamin C from 60 mg to at least 100–200 mg per day. This same panel also cautioned that taking more than 1,000 mg of vitamin C daily could have adverse effects and recommended that "whenever possible, vitamin C intake should come from fruits and vegetables"—more support for getting at least your "daily five" servings of fruits and vegetables.

Although the Food and Nutrition Board has recently raised the RDA for vitamin C from 60 mg to 75–90 mg (instead of to 100–200 mg per day, as recommended by the expert panel), it is well established that almost everybody can benefit from even higher levels. For example, the vitamin C recommendation for cigarette smokers is 100–200 mg per day, because smoking destroys vitamin C in the body. You need not worry about developing scurvy (as long as you consume at least 10 mg of vitamin C daily), but be sure to increase your intake if you're exposed to stress (physical or psychological) or infection (for example from a sick friend of family member).

In terms of safety, vitamin C is extremely safe even at relatively high doses, because most of the excess is excreted in the urine. At high doses (over 1,000 mg per day), however, some people experience gastrointestinal side effects such as stomach cramps, nausea, and diarrhea. In addition, vitamin C intakes above 1,000 mg per day may increase the risk of developing kidney stones in some people.

Although vitamin C is well absorbed, the percentage absorbed from supplements decreases with higher dosages; therefore, optimal absorption is achieved by taking several small doses throughout the day. For example, try 100–250 mg per dose for a total daily intake of 250–1,000 mg. Full blood and tissue saturation is typically achieved with intakes of 250–500 mg per day.

Sharon was a high-achieving college student who experienced an extreme degree of anxiety and stress during exams—particularly during midterm and final-exam periods. Like millions of students around the world, Sharon was far more likely to become sick (usually catching a cold or the flu) during exam periods than at other times of the year. During exam periods, the combination of poor diet (lots of junk food), inadequate sleep (late-night study sessions), and heightened anxiety (about grades) led to a cortisol-induced suppression of immune-system function—and a dramatic rise in illness rates for Sharon and her classmates.

To guard against the inevitable increase in cortisol levels and suppression of immune function during midterm-exam week, Sharon supplemented her diet with a cortisol-controlling blend of vitamin C (250 mg, taken twice daily) and phytosterols (60 mg of beta-sitosterol, taken twice daily), along with a direct immune-boosting dose of echinacea (125 mg, taken twice daily). (For more about phytosterols and echinacea, see Chapters 8 and 11, respectively.) Unfortunately, she also kept up her steady pre-exam diet of Mountain Dew, M&M's, and inadequate sleep. Despite this less than optimal foundation of diet and sleep for controlling cortisol levels, the supplement regimen appeared to bring Sharon's immune system through midterms with flying colors: She avoided catching a cold during or after her exams this year.

CALCIUM

Calcium is the most abundant mineral in the human body, and although 99 percent of your body's calcium is stored in the bones, the remaining 1 percent is found in the blood and within cells, where it performs a vital role in dozens of metabolic processes. Research into the effects of calcium on metabolism has revealed the profound impact of calcium in such areas as reducing your risk of colon cancer, cutting symptoms of PMS in half (pain, bloating, mood swings, and food cravings), and controlling blood pressure. If that weren't enough evidence that calcium supplements might be a good idea, there is also some evidence that calcium can even influence mood and behavior. This possibility comes from studies of rats in which the animals become agitated when fed a low-calcium diet, but are more calm and relaxed when their diets contain adequate calcium levels.

As a dietary supplement, calcium is about as safe as it gets, with side effects being quite rare and modest in severity (occasional constipation at higher intakes). Because practically nobody consumes enough calcium in their daily diet, and with calcium being so cheap and easily available, this is certainly one of the nutrients for which supplementation is highly recommended.

MAGNESIUM

Magnesium is a mineral that functions as a coenzyme (the active part of an enzyme system) for nerve and muscle function, regulation of body temperature, energy metabolism, DNA and RNA synthesis, and the formation of bones. The majority of the body's magnesium (60 percent) is found in the bones; therefore, many of us tend to think of magnesium as a bone-specific nutrient.

Because magnesium serves as a cofactor for so many regulatory enzymes, particularly those involved with energy metabolism and nervous-system function, magnesium needs may increase during periods of heightened stress. Magnesium is required for proper enzyme function in converting carbohydrates, protein, and fat into energy—and at least a few studies have suggested a potential role for magnesium supplements in energy metabolism by showing increased exercise efficiency in endurance athletes. Although there is no overwhelming evidence to suggest any increases in muscular strength or elevated energy levels following magnesium supplementation, clinical studies have shown magnesium supplements to help lessen feelings of anxiety and overall stress.

The Daily Value (DV, another term for RDA) for magnesium is 400 mg per day, but requirements may be elevated somewhat by stressors such as exercise. Additionally, because magnesium increases calcium absorption, it is recommended that calcium supplements taken for bone building or prevention of bone loss contain magnesium. Food sources include artichokes, nuts, beans, whole grains, and shellfish, but since nearly three-quarters of the American population fails to consume enough magnesium, supplements may be warranted—especially during periods of heightened stress. Excessive magnesium intake can cause diarrhea and general gastrointestinal distress, as well as interfere with calcium absorption and bone metabolism (even though optimal levels of magnesium *assist* calcium absorption). Therefore, since no known benefits are associated with consuming more than 600 mg per day of magnesium, higher intakes should be avoided.

THIAMIN

Thiamin, also known as vitamin B-1, is a water-soluble vitamin that functions in carbohydrate metabolism to help convert pyruvate to acetyl CoA for entry into the Krebs cycle and subsequent steps to generate ATP. All this is technical talk for saying that thiamin helps give you energy. Thiamin also functions in maintaining the health of the nervous system and heart muscle. Food sources of thiamin include nuts, liver, brewer's yeast, and pork.

Because of thiamin's role in carbohydrate metabolism and nerve function, supplements have been promoted for increasing energy levels and maintaining memory. Thiamin also seems to be involved in the release of the neurotransmitter acetylcholine from nerve cells, and thiamin deficiency is associated with generalized muscle weakness and mental confusion.

Dietary thiamin requirements are based on caloric intake, so individuals who consume more calories, such as athletes, are likely to require a higher than average intake of thiamin to help process the extra carbohydrates into energy. During acute periods of stress, thiamin needs may be temporarily elevated, but outright thiamin deficiencies are rare except in individuals consuming a severely restricted diet.

No adverse side effects are known with thiamin intakes at RDA levels or even at levels several times the RDA, which is 1.5 mg. Virtually every multivitamin contains thiamin at 100 percent RDA levels or higher—with supplements focused on alleviating stress containing two to ten times RDA levels, which are still quite safe.

RIBOFLAVIN

Riboflavin, also known as vitamin B-2, is a water-soluble vitamin that serves primarily as a coenzyme for many metabolic processes in the body, such as formation of red blood cells and function of the nervous system. Riboflavin is involved in energy production as part of the electron transport chain that produces cellular energy. As a building block for FAD (flavin adenine dinucleotide), riboflavin is a crucial component in converting food into energy. FAD is required for electron transport and ATP production in the Krebs cycle. Liver, dairy products, dark-green vegetables, and many seafoods are good sources of riboflavin.

Requirements for riboflavin, like most B vitamins, are related to calorie intake—so the more food you eat, the more riboflavin you need to support the metabolic processes that will convert the food into usable energy (but by eating the right foods, such as dairy products and veggies, you'll also be getting more riboflavin as well). Women should be aware that riboflavin needs are elevated during pregnancy and lactation, as well as by the use of oral contraceptives (birth-control pills). Athletes may require more riboflavin due to both increased caloric intake and increased needs from exercise, which the body perceives as a stressor.

There is no strong support for the efficacy of isolated riboflavin supplements in promoting health outside of correcting a nutrient deficiency. Despite the role of riboflavin in a variety of energy-generating processes, the chances of a supplement's improving energy levels in a well-nourished person is unlikely, but those individuals under high levels of emotional or physical stress may have increased requirements.

No serious side effects have been reported for supplementation with riboflavin at levels several times above the DV of 1.7 mg. Because the body excretes excess riboflavin in the urine, high supplemental levels are likely to result in fluorescent-yellow urine.

PANTOTHENIC ACID

Pantothenic acid, also known as vitamin B-5, is a water-soluble vitamin widely distributed in most animal and plant foods. It is physiologically active as part of two coenzymes: acetyl coenzyme A (CoA) and acyl carrier protein. Pantothenic acid functions in the oxidation of fatty acids and carbohydrates for energy production, as well as in the synthesis of fatty acids, ketones, cholesterol, phospholipids, steroid hormones, and amino acids. Food sources include liver, egg yolk, fresh vegetables, legumes, yeast, and whole grains. Because it is found in many foods, a deficiency is extremely rare in people who consume a varied diet.

Vitamin B-5 is often referred to as an "antistress" vitamin because of its central role in adrenal-cortex function and cellular metabolism. Unfortunately, there is limited evidence from controlled studies to suggest that pantothenic acid taken on its own will reduce feelings of stress and anxiety or provide protection during times of stress. Therefore, it probably makes more sense to consume vitamin B-5, along with the other B-complex vitamins, as part of a balanced blend of all the essential nutrients, because there is good cortisol-control data for mixtures of B vitamins that include B-5.

As a water-soluble B vitamin, B-5 is generally considered a safe supplement, but large doses (10 grams or more) may cause diarrhea. Additional supplementation beyond the levels found in a multivitamin blend (5–50 mg per day) is probably unnecessary.

PYRIDOXINE

Pyridoxine, also known as vitamin B-6, is a water-soluble vitamin that performs as a cofactor for about seventy different enzyme systems, most of which have something to do with amino-acid and protein metabolism. Because vitamin B-6 is also involved in the synthesis of neurotransmitters in the brain and nerve cells, it is frequently recommended as a nutrient to support mental function (mood) and nerve conduction, especially during periods of heightened stress. Some athletic supplements include vitamin B-6 because of its role in the conversion of glycogen to glucose for energy in muscle tissue. Food sources include poultry, fish, whole grains, and bananas.

Vitamin B-6, like most of the B vitamins, is involved as a cofactor in a wide variety of enzyme systems. As such, claims can be made for virtually any health condition. For example, because B-6 is needed in the conversion of the amino acid tryptophan into niacin, a common B-6 claim relates to healthy cholesterol levels, because niacin can help lower cholesterol in some people. Because B-6 also plays a role in prostaglandin synthesis, claims are often made for B-6 in regulating blood pressure, heart function, and pain levels, each of which is partially regulated by prostaglandins. Vitamin B-6 needs are increased in individuals consuming a high-protein diet, as well as in women taking oral contraceptives (birth-control pills).

Vitamin B-6 supplements, in conjunction with folic acid, have been shown to have a significant effect in reducing plasma levels of homocysteine (an amino acid metabolite linked to increased risk of atherosclerosis). In many animal models of hypertension, supplemental pyridoxine lowers blood pressure, and there is pre-liminary evidence for antihypertensive activity in humans as well. Additionally, we know that physiological levels of pyridoxal phosphate (PLP, the active form of B-6) interact with glucocorticoid (cortisol) receptors to down-regulate their activity—suggesting that B-6 supplements may be able to favorably counteract some of the adverse effects of elevated cortisol levels.

Numerous animal studies have shown that animals subjected to various stressors have an increased incidence of gastric ulcers. Animals supplemented with pyridoxine tend to have fewer stress-induced ulcers compared to animals given placebo. In one notable study of rabbits exposed to hypoxic stress (resulting from high alti-tude and reduced oxygen levels), pyridoxine feeding was shown to reduce plasma levels of cortisol by as much as 55 percent.

As a water-soluble B vitamin, pyridoxine is generally very safe as a dietary supplement. Excessive intakes (2–6 grams acutely or

500 mg chronically) are associated with sensory neuropathy (loss of feeling in the extremities), which may or may not be reversible. The RDA for vitamin B-6 is only 2 mg per day, an amount contained in virtually all multivitamin supplements. Pregnant and lactating women should not take more than 100 mg of vitamin B-6 per day.

Summary

When it comes to dietary supplementation for stress adaptation and cortisol control, the first line of defense appears in the form of a comprehensive multivitamin/multimineral supplement. The most effective choices will be those products that offer a balanced blend of the key vitamins and minerals the body needs during the stress response. In particular, vitamin C, magnesium, and the full B-complex group are probably most important from the standpoint of their direct involvement in the body's stress response, but all of the essential and semiessential vitamins and trace minerals are needed as well. A comprehensive multivitamin/multimineral supplement, when used as part of a regimen of balanced diet and regular exercise, represents the antistress foundation on which you can add the targeted cortisol-control supplements that are covered in chapters to come.

. . . .
                    .
                    .
                    .

CHAPTER 8

Cortisol-Control
Supplements

The preceding chapter outlined the importance for everybody of establishing a sound antistress foundation with a balanced multivitamin supplement. For some people, that general nutrition foundation will be enough to help control cortisol and the stress response. For most others, however, a more targeted cortisol-controlling supplementation regimen may be needed to directly modulate the stress response and control cortisol levels within a healthy range.

For example, the Stressed Jesses among us will certainly need a *daily* cortisol-control regimen—and they'll need to follow it very closely. Strained Janes will also benefit from their own cortisol-control regimen, but they have the luxury of being somewhat less strict, so missing a day of cortisol control is not the end of the world. Relaxed Jack might only need to think about controlling his cortisol levels on an infrequent basis, such as during the rare times when he is under heightened stress. This chapter outlines some of the most promising supplements for directly modulating the stress response and helping to bring cortisol levels into a more healthful range.

MAGNOLIA BARK

Magnolia bark (*Magnolia officinalis*) is a traditional Chinese medicine (in China it is known as *houpu* or *hou po*) used since A.D. 100 for treating stagnation of *qi* (low energy) as well as a variety of syndromes, such as digestive disturbances caused by emotional distress and emotional turmoil. Magnolia bark is rich in two biphenol compounds, magnolol and honokiol, which are thought to contribute to the primary antistress and cortisol-lowering effects of the plant. The magnolol content of magnolia bark is generally in the range of 2–10 percent, while honokiol tends to occur naturally at 1–5 percent in dried magnolia bark. Magnolia bark also contains a bit less than 1 percent of an essential oil known as *eudesmol*, which is classified as a triterpene compound, and may provide some additional benefits as an antioxidant.

Two of the most popular herbal medicines used in Japan, one called *saiboku-to* and another called *hange-kobuku-to*, contain magnolia bark and have been used for treating ailments from bronchial asthma to depression to anxiety. Japanese researchers have determined that the magnolol and honokiol components of *Magnolia officinalis* are one thousand times more potent than alpha-tocopherol (vitamin E) in their antioxidant activity, thereby offering a potential heart-health benefit. Other research groups have shown both magnolol and honokiol to possess powerful "brain-health" benefits via their actions in modulating the activity of various neurotransmitters and related enzymes in the brain (increased choline acetyltransferase activity, inhibition of acetylcholinesterase, and increased acetylcholine release).

Numerous animal studies have demonstrated that honokiol acts as a central-nervous-system depressant at high doses, but as a nonsedating anxiolytic (antianxiety and antistress) agent at lower doses. This means that a small dose of honokiol, or a magnolia bark extract standardized for honokiol content, can help to destress a person without making her sleepy, while a larger dose might have the effect of knocking her out. When compared to pharmaceutical agents such as Valium (diazepam), honokiol appears to be as effective in its antianxiety activity, yet not nearly as powerful in its sedative ability. These results have been demonstrated in at least half a dozen animal studies and suggest that magnolia-bark extracts standardized for honokiol content would be an appropriate approach for controlling the detrimental effects of everyday stressors without the tranquilizing side effects of pharmaceutical agents.

No significant toxicity or adverse effects have been associated with traditional use of magnolia bark, which is as a decoction (hot-water tea) using 3–9 grams of dried bark (and only obtained via a practitioner of traditional Chinese medicine). Extracts of magnolia bark are now available in commercial antianxiety products; these come in a powdered or pill form at doses of 250–750 mg per day and standardized to 1–2 percent honokiol and magnolol.

> *Rachel,* the single mom in Chapter 4 who suffered from stress-related irritability and anxiety, was an avid fitness walker and vegetarian. As such, she already had the diet and exercise part of her cortisol-control regimen well covered. By adding a twice-daily supplement of magnolia bark extract (150 mg in the A.M. and 300 mg in the P.M.), she was able to reduce a great deal of her perceived stress, anxiety, and irritability. Rachel reported feeling more "balanced" and relaxed, but with no feelings of the drowsiness that is sometimes reported with drug-based antistress solutions.

THEANINE

Theanine is an amino acid found in the leaves of green tea (*Camellia sinensis*). Theanine offers quite different benefits from those imparted by the polyphenol and catechin antioxidants for which green tea is typically consumed. In fact, through the natural production of polyphenols, the tea plant converts theanine into catechins. This means tea leaves harvested during one part of the growing season may be high in catechins (good for antioxidant benefits), while leaves harvested during another time of year may be higher in theanine (good for antistress and cortisol-controlling effects). Theanine is unique in that it acts as a nonsedating relaxant to help increase the brain's production of alpha waves. This makes theanine extremely effective for combating tension, stress, and anxiety—without inducing drowsiness. Clinical studies show that theanine is effective in dosages ranging from 50–200 mg per day. Three to four cups of green tea are expected to contain 100–200 mg of theanine.

In addition to being considered a relaxing substance (in adults), theanine has also been shown to provide benefits for improving learning performance (in mice), and promoting concentration (in students). No adverse side effects are associated with theanine consumption, making it one of the leading natural choices for promoting relaxation without the sedating effects of depressant drugs and herbs. When considering the potential benefits of theanine as an antistress or anticortisol supplement, it is important to distinguish its nonsedating relaxation benefits from the tranquilizing effects of other relaxing supplements such as valerian and kava, which are actually mild central-nervous-system depressants.

As mentioned above, one of the most distinctive aspects of theanine activity is its ability to increase the brain's output of alpha waves. Alpha waves are one of the four basic brain-wave patterns (delta, theta, alpha, and beta) that can be monitored using an electroencephalogram (EEG). Each wave pattern is associated with a particular oscillating electrical voltage in the brain, and the different brain-wave patterns are associated with different mental states and states of consciousness (see Table 8.1).

Alpha waves, which indicate relaxed alertness, are nonexistent during deep sleep and during states of very high arousal such as fear or anger. During deep sleep, the predominant brain waves are the slow delta waves (0–4 cycles/second). When we are in light sleep, or merely drowsy, the slightly faster theta waves are the most prevalent (4–8 cycles/second). Beta waves, with the fastest cycle rates at 13–40 cycles/second, appear during highly stressful situations, when most of us find it difficult to concentrate or focus on anything. Alpha waves, at 8–13 cycles/second, are slower than high-stress beta waves, but faster than the delta/theta waves associated with sleep. They are the predominant brainwave pattern seen during wakefulness, when a person is engaged in relaxed and effortless alertness. In other words, alpha waves are associated with your highest levels of physical and mental performance; therefore, you want to maximize the amount of time during your waking hours that your brain spends in an alpha state.

An interesting analogy for emphasizing the importance of the different types of brain waves is to compare them to the gears of a car: The slowest brain waves (delta and theta) represent the "idling" and "getting started" gears, alpha acts as the primary "working gear," and beta functions as the fastest "hyperdrive" gear, where you might be spinning your wheels instead of getting anywhere. Just as you use different gears in your car for different driving conditions, your brain generates different wave patterns when it is engaged in different activities. For example, too few theta and delta waves means that you're likely to suffer from insomnia, while too many would cause you to stumble around in a constant drowsy fog. The best situation is to experience an orderly process from one brain-wave pattern to the next—from restful sleep (delta/theta) to focused alertness (alpha) and back to restful sleep (theta/delta)—throughout a twenty-four-hour period. You'll notice that beta has been left out of the ideal cycle, because we don't need to experience anger or agitation if we can avoid it.

Unfortunately, our high-stress modern lifestyles result in the majority of us skipping our second and third brain gears (theta and alpha). Many people wake up suddenly out of a deep sleep (delta) with an alarm clock, which induces immediate stress and anxiety (beta) about being late or being under time pressure. After insufficient sleep, we use stimulants (caffeine) to force us into an artificial wakefulness that promotes beta waves (and higher cortisol levels) while suppressing both theta and alpha waves (and inhibiting cortisol reduction). For much of the day, the combined effects

Table 8.1: Brain-Wave Oscillation Patterns

Brain-Wave Pattern	Cycles per Second	Mood/State of Consciousness
Delta	0–4	Deep sleep (stages 3 and 4)
Theta	4–8	Drowsy/light sleep (stages 1 and 2)
Alpha	8–13	Relaxed/wakeful/alert
Beta	13–40	Stressed/anxious/difficulty concentrating

of work stress and time urgency have us swimming in beta waves and high cortisol levels. By the time we finally get to bed at night, we're so exhausted that we completely bypass the unwinding benefits of theta sleep (when cortisol levels fall) and instead fall unconscious into the deeper (delta) stages of sleep, but rarely for long enough.

Why is all this talk about brain waves important? Because this constant charging back and forth between delta and beta brain waves tends to keep cortisol levels elevated throughout the daylight hours (a bad thing) while also disallowing time for those levels to subside during the night (a *really* bad thing). In terms of our mental and physical performance, a constant lack of theta and alpha waves means that we can't concentrate (alpha) when we need to, and we can't relax (theta) when we want to.

And this is where theanine comes in. By increasing the brain's output of alpha waves, theanine can help us to "rebalance" our brain-wave patterns, as well as help to control anxiety, increase focus and concentration, promote creativity, and improve our overall mental and physical performance. Research studies are quite clear on the facts that people who produce more alpha brain waves also have less anxiety; that highly creative people generate more alpha waves when faced with a problem to solve; and that elite athletes tend to produce a burst of alpha waves on the left side of their brain during their best performances.

Pretty good stuff—and the best way to increase your output of alpha waves is via theanine consumption. This can easily be accomplished by consuming three to four cups of green tea each day (theanine counteracts a fair portion of the stimulant effect of caffeine), or by taking a daily theanine supplement (50–200 mg per day). Before you decide to use decaffeinated green tea as a source of theanine, be aware that most of the theanine is lost during the decaffeination process, so if you wish to avoid caffeine entirely, a supplement may be your most reliable source. Theanine supplements are available in capsule or tablet form as pure (synthetic) theanine, and as a natural extract from green tea (enriched to as much as 20–35 percent theanine). Because theanine reaches its maximum levels in the blood between thirty minutes and two hours after taking it, it can be used both as a daily cortisol-control regimen and "as needed" during stressful events.

EPIMEDIUM

Epimedium is a genus of twenty-one related plant species. The Chinese refer to epimedium as *yin yang huo*, which can be loosely translated as "licentious goat plant" and explains why Western supplement companies have adopted the titillating name by which it is known in the United States: horny goat weed. Epimedium is grown as an ornamental herb in Asia and the Mediterranean region, and various species are used for medicinal purposes, including *Epimedium sagittatum, Epimedium brevicornum, Epimedium wushanense, Epimedium koreanum,* and *Epimedium pubescens.*

The use of epimedium as a medicinal herb dates back to at least A.D. 400. It has been used as a tonic for the reproductive system (boosting libido and treating impotence) and as a rejuvenating tonic (to relieve fatigue). Animal studies have shown that epimedium may function a bit like an adaptogen (more on adaptogens appears in the next chapter) by increasing levels of epinephrine, norepinephrine, serotonin, and dopamine when they are low (an energy-promoting effect), but reducing cortisol levels when they are elevated (an antistress effect). There is also evidence that epimedium can restore low levels of both testosterone and thyroid hormone to their normal levels; this may account for some of the benefits of epimedium in improving libido (sex drive). Animal studies using epimedium have shown a reduction in bone breakdown, an increase in muscle mass, and a loss of body fat— each of which may be linked to the observed reduction of elevated cortisol down to normal levels.

In a series of studies conducted in humans and animals by Chinese researchers, immune-system function was directly suppressed and bone loss was accelerated by using high-dose synthetic cortisol (glucocorticoid drugs). Subsequent administration of epimedium extract reduced blood levels of cortisol and improved immune-system function (in the humans) and slowed bone loss and strengthened bones (in the animals).

It is interesting to note that although at least fifteen active compounds have been identified in epimedium extracts (luteolin, icariin, quercetin, and various epimedins), many supplement companies currently use extracts standardized only for icariin. The traditional use of epimedium is as a hot-water decoction (tea), which would result in a very different profile of active constituents when compared to the high-icariin alcohol extracts that are more commonly used in commercial products. Although at least one test-tube study has shown icariin to protect liver cells from damage by various toxic compounds, other feeding studies (in rodents) have suggested that high-dose icariin may be associated with kidney and liver toxicity.

Because all of the existing scientific evidence for the antistress and cortisol-controlling effect of epimedium has been demonstrated for water-extracted epimedium (that is, as a tea), and because this form of extraction may result in a safer form of epimedium (compared to the high-icariin alcohol extract), it may be prudent to select supplements that specifically use a more traditional formulation. Commercial preparations of the water-extracted form of epimedium will indicate on their labels that they are water-extracted, while the more concentrated (high-icariin) alcohol extracts tend to emphasize their icariin content (usually

20 percent or so). There have been no reports of adverse side effects associated with the traditional, water-extracted preparation of epimedium at the suggested dosage (250–1,000 mg per day for cortisol control).

> You may remember *Holly* and *Alan* from Chapter 4 as the young newlyweds whose high-achievement, high-stress lives resulted in a disconcerting loss of libido. Both exercised religiously (four to five times each week), but their diets needed some tweaking; specifically, each needed a better balance of carbs with proteins, more fresh fruits and veggies, and to adopt more regular eating patterns. Along with these nutritional recommendations, they both started on a supplement regimen of epimedium (300 mg per day) and DHEA (25 mg per day for Holly and 50 mg per day for Alan). For more about DHEA see Chapter 11.
>
> After about one week on the supplements, Holly and Alan were grinning from ear to ear (we need not go into the details why). The combination of epimedium and DHEA helped to normalize their cortisol-to-DHEA ratios as well as their libidos, and helped to put the spark back in their sex life.

PHYTOSTEROLS

Phytosterols include hundreds of plant-derived sterol compounds (including sterols and sterolins) that bear structural similarity to the cholesterol made in our bodies, but none of the artery-clogging effects. The most prevalent phytosterols in the diet are beta-sitosterol (BS), campesterol, and stigmasterol. Plant oils contain the highest concentration of phytosterols, so nuts and seeds have fairly high levels, and all fruits and vegetables generally contain some. Perhaps the best way to obtain phytosterols is to eat a diet rich in fruits, vegetables, nuts, and seeds—which obviously would bring numerous other benefits as well.

Phytosterols appear to help modulate immune function, inflammation, and pain levels through their effects on controlling the production of inflammatory cytokines. This modulation of cytokine production and activity may also help to control allergies and reduce prostate enlargement. In athletes competing in marathons and other endurance events, phytosterols are known to reduce cortisol levels, maintain DHEA levels, and prevent the typical suppression of immune-system function seen after endurance events. From test-tube and animal studies, it appears that phytosterols such as beta-sitosterol can influence the structure and function of cell membranes in both healthy and cancerous tissue. This effect is known to alter cellular signaling pathways that regulate tumor growth and apoptosis (cell death); it provides a possible explanation for the stimulation of immune function observed following beta-sitosterol supplementation.

In several animal studies examining the effect of beta-sitosterol consumption on experimentally induced breast cancer, the animals fed phytosterols (including beta-sitosterol) showed a dramatic (30–80 percent) reduction in tumor size and a 10–30 percent lower incidence of metastases to the lymph nodes and lungs compared to a control group. From these animal studies, there is strong preliminary evidence that dietary phytosterols do indeed retard the growth and spread of breast cancer cells.

In terms of general immune function, beta-sitosterol has been shown in humans to normalize the function of T-helper lymphocytes and natural killer cells following stressful events, such as marathon running, that normally suppress immune-system function. In addition to alleviating much of the postexercise immune suppression that occurs following endurance competitions, beta-sitosterol has also been shown to normalize the ratio of catabolic stress hormones (i.e., those that break down tissue, such as cortisol) to anabolic (rebuilding) hormones such as DHEA.

In one small study, seventeen endurance runners completed a sixty-eight-kilometer run (about forty miles) and afterward received either 60 mg of beta-sitosterol (nine runners) or a placebo (eight runners) for four weeks. Those runners receiving the beta-sitosterol supplements showed a significant drop in their cortisol-to-DHEA ratio (indicating less stress) as well as reduced inflammation and a markedly lower immunosuppression. Using the ultramarathon as a model for overall stress, researchers concluded that beta-sitosterol is effective in modulating the stress response by managing cortisol levels within a more normal range.

Phytosterols are generally regarded as quite safe because of their widespread distribution in fruits and vegetables. No significant side effects or drug interactions have been reported in any of the studies investigating beta-sitosterol. The typical dosage recommended to achieve the best cortisol-control and immune-function benefits is 100–300 mg per day of a mixed phytosterol blend, including 60–120 mg per day of beta-sitosterol. A handful of roasted peanuts or a couple of tablespoons of peanut butter contain about 10–30 mg of beta-sitosterol, so a few handfuls of Planter's nuts or a scoop of Skippy will supply an effective dose of immune enhancement following exercise (but also a whopping dose of calories).

Because phytosterols have other health benefits in addition to their role in cortisol control, they are often found in commercial supplements for lowering cholesterol (several margarine-like spreads), boosting immune function (tablets and capsules), and maintaining prostate health (tablets and capsules). Almost always, the phytosterols will be combined with additional ingredients to enhance the primary effect (for example, they might be blended with echinacea in immune-boosting products).

PHOSPHATIDYLSERINE

Phosphatidylserine (PS) is a phospholipid—meaning that it is composed of fatty acids (lipids) and phosphate. PS is concentrated in the brain cells, where it is thought to be related to brain-cell function, but it is also found in *all* cell membranes, where it is thought to play key roles in muscle metabolism and immune-system function. PS has also been shown to modulate many aspects of cortisol overproduction, especially following intense exercise.

There is ample scientific evidence that PS supplementation, in a dose of 100–300 mg per day, can help improve mental function and depression, even in cases as severe as Alzheimer's disease and other forms of age-related mental decline. More recent studies from Italy have shown larger doses of PS (400–800 mg per day) to reduce cortisol levels by 15–30 percent following heavy exercise. Because cortisol is catabolic toward muscle tissue (that is, it leads to protein breakdown and muscle loss), athletes frequently use PS supplements to help promote recovery from exercise and help slow muscle loss. And because of its benefits in improving cognitive function, PS could also be considered a general anti-stress nutrient, providing benefits not only for athletes subjected to the physical stress of exercise, but also for individuals who are under chronic emotional stress from hectic lifestyles, job deadlines, and many of the other stresses of a modern, Type C lifestyle.

There do not appear to be any significant side effects associated with dietary supplements containing phosphatidylserine, but due to concerns about mad-cow disease, it is generally recommended to select PS supplements derived from soybeans versus those extracted from cows' brains.

Concentrated PS supplements are available in doses of 50–100 mg per day, and they are quite expensive. For brain and mental support, 100–500 mg per day of PS is recommended for a month or so, followed by a lower maintenance dose of approximately 50–100 mg per day. Athletes may need as much as 800 mg per day immediately before or following intense training to help suppress cortisol secretion and promote muscle recovery. This amount of PS would cost several hundred dollars per month, making these levels less than viable for the average consumer.

Ken was an avid runner, regularly competing in 10K races and occasional marathons. Frustrated with his apparent inability to fully recover between strenuous workouts and intense competitions, despite a regimen of active rest and balanced nutrition, Ken turned to a combination of supplements that included phosphatidylserine (PS) and beta-sitosterol (BS). Both PS and

BS have been shown to help athletes reduce the rise in cortisol that is seen during intense exercise. Because elevated cortisol levels are catabolic toward connective tissues such as muscle, tendons, and ligaments—that is, they accelerate the breakdown of these tissues—keeping cortisol levels from rising too high during exercise can be an effective strategy for reducing tissue breakdown and enhancing the repair process.

The combination of PS (50 mg per day) with BS (200 mg per day), taken immediately following each workout, helped Ken's body to control cortisol levels and accelerate his postexercise recovery. The primary end benefit for Ken was a heightened ability to train intensely without getting injured and, thus, to improve his overall performance in his races.

TYROSINE

Tyrosine is an amino acid that has been studied by the U.S. military as a potential antistress nutrient to help soldiers cope with the stress of battle. Findings from several studies suggest that dietary tyrosine supplements can help to reduce the acute effects of stress and fatigue on physical and mental performance. Chronic stress can reduce brain levels of neurotransmitters such as epinephrine, norepinephrine, and dopamine, a phenomenon thought to be related to some of the decline in mental and physical performance during stressful events. Because the brain uses tyrosine to synthesize these neurotransmitters, dietary tyrosine supplements can help slow their depletion and reduce the declines in performance that are often noted during stressful events. And because neurotransmitters play a role in overall brain function, including depression and other mood disorders, tyrosine supplementation has been studied for its effects on stress, mental function, and Alzheimer's disease.

In soldiers, this theory has been proven under conditions of combat training, sleep deprivation, cold exposure, and extremes of physical exercise. Studies of military cadets undergoing combat training showed that 2,000 mg of tyrosine aided memory and cognitive ability during stress. In other (nonsoldier) studies, tyrosine supplements (100–200 mg per day) were able to offset declines in performance and ability to concentrate in volunteers exposed to stressful situations such as shift work, sleep deprivation, and fatigue.

In animals, dietary tyrosine supplementation has been shown to improve learning ability and memory (ability to navigate a maze), while tyrosine depletion has led to decreased performance, probably via suppressed norepinephrine levels. Tyrosine and norepinephrine levels are often reduced in people with depression or under conditions of stress, and in some forms of obesity. In animal experiments, tyrosine supplementation leads to a slight elevation in oxygen consumption, suggesting an effect on increasing metabolic rate.

In one human study, 6–8 grams of tyrosine or a placebo was given to volunteers subjected to a cardiovascular stress test. Those receiving the tyrosine supplements showed improvements in attention and cognitive function compared to the placebo group. In another study, subjects were given either a placebo or 6–7 grams of tyrosine, in random order on two consecutive days. One hour later, subjects were asked to perform a number of stress-sensitive tasks while simultaneously being exposed to a stressor (loud noise). During the tyrosine supplementation, subjects showed improved performance and decreased blood pressure throughout the study period. In an additional double-blind, placebo-controlled crossover study, subjects receiving 6–7 grams of tyrosine showed a significant improvement in stress symptoms, mood disturbances, and performance impairments during exposure to extreme stress (four and a half hours of cold and low oxygen). Overall, these studies suggest that tyrosine is effective in modulating the stress response in a variety of stressful conditions.

Since tyrosine is relatively abundant in protein-containing foods, it is unlikely that tyrosine supplements in the levels commonly available would cause significant side effects. Human studies have been conducted with 6–8 grams of tyrosine per day, with no adverse effects noted. (Because of the high cost of tyrosine supplements, commercially available products tend to provide no more than a few hundred milligrams—that is, less than 10 percent of the levels shown to be effective against stress in clinical studies.) Extremely high doses of any isolated amino acid are not recommended, however, as they may cause unpleasant gastrointestinal side effects such as diarrhea, nausea, and vomiting, as well as headaches and nervousness.

BRANCHED-CHAIN AMINO ACIDS

The group of amino acids referred to as the *branched-chain amino acids* (BCAAs) is comprised of three essential amino acids: valine, leucine, and isoleucine. The recommended intake for the BCAAs is about 3 grams per day, an amount that should be easily obtained from protein foods. Supplemental levels have been used at doses from 3 grams to more than 20 grams per day to increase endurance, reduce fatigue, improve mental performance, increase energy levels, prevent immune-system suppression, and counteract muscle catabolism following intense exercise.

In numerous studies of athletes, BCAAs have been shown to maintain blood levels of glutamine, an amino acid used as fuel by immune-system cells. During intense exercise, glutamine levels typically fall dramatically, removing the primary fuel source for immune cells and leading to a general suppression of immune-system activity (and an increased risk of infections) following the exercise. By supplementing with either glutamine or BCAA, a person can maintain blood levels of glutamine and thereby avoid suppression of immune-cell activity due to a lack of fuel.

In related studies, BCAA supplements have been shown to bear a beneficial effect on counteracting the rise in cortisol and the drop in testosterone that is often seen in endurance athletes undergoing stressful training. In these studies, intense exercise is used as a model for high stress, so the increased cortisol levels and the reduced testosterone levels are exactly what happen in the rest of us when we experience a stressful situation at work, at home, or in line at the grocery store.

Table 8.2: Dietary Supplements to Directly
Control Cortisol Levels: An Overview

Supplement	Benefits	Drawbacks	Overall Rank
Magnolia bark	Cortisol control and general effects as an antianxiety and antistress agent	Too much could cause sedation and drowsiness	Primary
Theanine	Modulates brain waves for optimal physical and mental performance during stressful events	None	Primary
Epimedium	Direct cortisol control, especially following the stress of dieting	Alcohol extract may be toxic; choose a water extract	Primary
Phytosterols	Balances cortisol-to-DHEA ratio, especially following exercise stress	None	Primary
Phos-phatidylserine (PS)	Direct cortisol-lowering effect, especially after intense exercise	High cost at effective doses	Secondary
Tyrosine	Maintains mental perform-ance and concentration during stressful events	High doses needed	Secondary
Branched-chain amino acids (BCAAs)	Reduce muscle breakdown and immune suppression during exercise stress	High doses needed	Secondary

Supplemental intakes of the BCAAs (3–20 grams per day) have been studied in tablet and liquid form with no reported adverse side effects, aside from minor gastrointestinal complaints. Higher intakes should be avoided due to the possibility of blocking the absorption of other amino acids from the diet and the risk of more severe gastrointestinal distress. Unfortunately, because purified sources of the BCAAs are so expensive, commercial products typically provide only a small fraction of the multigram doses that have been studied for performance and recovery.

Summary

The seven supplements discussed in this chapter—magnolia bark, theanine, epimedium, phytosterols, phosphatidylserine, tyrosine, and BCAAs—represent the most promising natural compounds for directly controlling stress and modulating cortisol levels. But which of them should you choose? One? Three? All seven? To narrow down your choices, it may be helpful to refer to Table 8.2 on the previous page.

. . . .
.
.
.

CHAPTER 9

Adaptogens (General Antistress Supplements)

O ne of the primary traditional approaches to dealing with chronic stress involves the use of a class of herbs referred to collectively as *adaptogens*. These herbs—most notably ginseng, ashwagandha, schisandra, rhodiola, astragalus, suma, and several Asian mushrooms (reishi, maitake, and shiitake)—are thought to alleviate many symptoms and side effects of chronic stress because they help to bring many metabolic systems back toward normal ranges. While the mechanisms of action for these antistress effects are not completely understood for most adaptogenic herbs (and for suma and the Asian mushrooms there is a lack of Western scientific evidence to support their centuries-old use for treating fatigue, anxiety, and stress), across the studies that *have* been conducted, it is clear that at least part of this adaptogenic response is due to effects of the herbs within the adrenal glands, the same place where cortisol is produced.

A variety of experiments have demonstrated similarities between the various adaptogenic herbs in affecting both the adrenal glands and the HPA axis. (Recall from earlier chapters that the HPA axis is the system of three hormonal glands that together mediate our response to stress.) In animal experiments, the range of compounds isolated from adaptogenic herbs appears to provide a "buffering" or "balancing" action that counteracts an exaggerated adrenal response to stress and reduces cortisol secretion back down toward normal levels, while also stimulating adrenal-gland activity during periods of fatigue and low energy levels.

GINSENG

Ginseng is perhaps the most potent (or at least the best known) of the adaptogens. A strain of ginseng known as *panax ginseng* (also called *Korean ginseng*) provides the most well-substantiated effects. Other forms, such as American and Siberian ginseng, contain some of the same compounds found in the Korean species, but in slightly different proportions that provide slightly different effects in terms of antistress benefits. Numerous animal and human studies show that ginseng can increase energy and endurance, improve mental function (learning and maze tests), and improve overall resistance to various stressors including viruses and bacteria, extreme exercise, and sleep deprivation. Human studies have shown improved immune function and reduced incidence of colds and flu following a month of supplementation with 100 mg per day of panax ginseng. In a handful of studies, ginseng has also provided benefits in terms of mental function in volunteers exposed to stress; improvements in ability to form abstract thoughts, in reaction times, and in scores on tests of memory and concentration were all evaluated following ginseng supplementation. In studies that measure general quality-of-life issues, ginseng supplementation at doses of 100–200 mg per day tends to result in improvements in mood, energy levels, stamina, and overall well-being.

In traditional Chinese medicine (TCM), panax ginseng is used as a tonic herb (a substance used to generally strengthen and invigorate the body) with adaptogenic properties (an adaptogen is a substance that helps one adapt to stressful situations). Some studies on ginseng have shown increased energy levels in fatigued subjects, but the majority of ginseng studies (mostly looking at athletic performance) have shown little to no effect. The differences between study results may be due to the fact that many commercially available ginseng supplements actually contain little or no ginseng at all, because the "real stuff" is very expensive.

Siberian ginseng (*Eleutherococcus senticosus; eleuthero* for short) is not truly ginseng, but it's a close enough cousin to deliver some of the same energetic benefits. Eleuthero is also known as *ciwujia* in popular sports/energy products. The Siberian form of ginseng is generally a less expensive alternative to Asian/Korean or panax ginseng, though it may have more of a stimulatory effect rather than an adaptogenic effect—not necessarily a bad thing if you just need a boost. Often promoted as an athletic-performance enhancer, eleuthero may also possess mild to moderate benefits in promoting recovery following intense exercise, perhaps due in part to an enhanced delivery of oxygen to recovering muscles.

The active compounds in ginseng are known as *ginsenosides*, and most of the top-quality ginseng supplements will be standardized for ginsenoside content. It is thought that the ginsenosides interact within the hypothalamic-pituitary-adrenal (HPA) axis to balance the body's secretion of adrenocorticotropic hormone (ACTH) and cortisol. ACTH has the ability to bind directly to brain cells and can affect a variety of stress-related processes in the body.

In general, 100–300 mg per day of properly standardized ginseng can improve general indices of stress and reduce the cortisol-to-DHEA ratio, which is a general gauge of overall stress. Ginseng is one of the many herbal supplements that can be purchased readily as a whole root, a dried powder, or a standardized extract. Because roots and powders can vary widely in their content of active compounds, the most precise approach to ensure that you are getting an effective product would be to use a standardized extract. It is also very important to select your ginseng supplement from a reliable manufacturer, as there are numerous examples of commercial products that provide little or no actual ginseng. Products should be standardized to contain 4–5 percent ginsenosides (for panax ginseng) or 0.5–1.0 percent eleutherosides (for Siberian ginseng). A daily intake of 100–300 mg for three to six weeks is recommended to produce adaptogenic and energetic benefits.

For the most part, plants in the ginseng family are generally considered to be quite safe. There are no known drug interactions, contraindications, common allergic reactions, or toxicity associated with Siberian ginseng, Panax ginseng, or American ginseng, although it is generally recommended that a course of treatment with ginseng not exceed three months. However, a word of caution is recommended for individuals with hypertension, as the stimulatory nature of some ginseng preparations has been reported to increase blood pressure. Additionally, individuals prone to hypoglycemia (low blood sugar) should use ginseng with caution due to the reported effects of ginseng to reduce blood-sugar levels.

ASHWAGANDHA

Ashwagandha (*Withania somnifera*) is an herb from India that is sometimes called *Indian ginseng*—not because it is part of the ginseng family, but to suggest similar energy-promoting and antistress benefits that are attributed to the more well known Asian and Siberian ginsengs. Although very little research has been done on ashwagandha, herbalists and natural-medicine practitioners often recommend the herb to combat stress and fatigue. Traditional use of ashwagandha in Indian (Ayurvedic) medicine is to "balance life forces" during stress and aging.

Commercial ashwagandha products are available in a variety of forms—from tablets and capsules to teas and liquids. Standardized powders provided as tablets or capsules generally provide the most stable and convenient dosage form. General dosage recommendations for ashwagandha range from 500–1,000 mg per day of an extract standardized to 1–2 percent withanolides, the herb's primary active component. Withanolides are thought to contribute to the calming effects of ashwagandha during periods of stress and may account for the use of ashwagandha as both a general tonic during stressful situations (where it is both calming and

fatigue fighting) and as a treatment for insomnia (where it promotes relaxation).

No long-term safety studies have been conducted on ashwagandha, but no reports of adverse side effects have been reported.
Because of the effects of ashwagandha on muscle relaxation and
as a mild central-nervous-system depressant, the herb should not
be combined with alcohol or other sedatives, sleep aids, or anxi-
olytics (antianxiety medications). Pregnant women are advised to
avoid ashwagandha due to its reported abortifacient (abortion-
inducing) effects and potential for premature labor.

> *Tracy* was a nurse in a critical-care hospital unit—and the long
> hours and irregular sleep schedule were beginning to wear her
> down. Strangely, despite her extreme level of fatigue when she
> eventually returned home each night, she had a great deal of
> trouble relaxing and falling asleep. Tracy tried several over-the-
> counter sleep remedies without much success, and she hated
> the hungover feeling they left her with the next morning. By
> incorporating a daily supplement of ashwagandha (150 mg in
> the A.M. and 300 mg in the P.M.), Tracy was able to control her
> feelings of stress while at work, without feeling sleepy, as well
> as to induce relaxation and restful sleep at night.

SUMA

Suma (*Pfaffia paniculata*) is a large ground vine native to Central
and South America; it is most notably from Brazil and often called
Brazilian ginseng. Traditional use of suma has been for improving
overall health and as a treatment for virtually every illness, leading to its native name of *para toda* (literally "for everything").
Modern recommendations for suma include claims of effects as an
adaptogen, an immune booster, and a treatment for chronic
fatigue and anxiety.

According to most contemporary herbalists, suma is best
understood as an adaptogen, a substance that helps one adapt to
stress and fight infection. Along with other adaptogens, such as
eleuthero, Russian Olympic athletes have used suma in the belief

that it will enhance sports performance. In the United States, suma is often recommended as a general strengthener of the body, as well as for treatment of chronic fatigue syndrome, ulcers, anxiety, impotence, and low resistance to illness—each of which is related to stress. Few studies have been conducted on suma, but those that are available (in animals) show an immune-strengthening and sexual-stimulation effect of suma, providing at least a small measure of support for the traditional use of the plant.

The typical dosage of suma is 500–1,000 mg per day during periods of heightened stress, anxiety, or fatigue. Suma is rarely found as a stand-alone commercial product, but is typically combined with other ingredients for targeting a specific condition (e.g., suma might be added to ginger and fiber to treat stress-induced ulcers).

SCHISANDRA

The fruit of the schisandra plant (*Schisandra chinensis*), also known as *wu-wei-wi* and sometimes spelled with a *z* (*schizandra*), has a long history of use in traditional Chinese medicine as an herb capable of promoting general well-being and enhancing vitality. In addition to its traditional uses for promoting energy and alleviating exhaustion and immune-system disturbances caused by stress, schisandra has historically been taken to strengthen the sex organs and promote mental function.

Schisandra is touted as a member of the adaptogen family, along with ginseng and related herbs, because of the presence of compounds thought to balance bodily functions related to stress. Lignans are a main constituent of schisandra and may be responsible for the herb's effects in stimulating the immune system, protecting the liver, increasing the body's ability to cope with stress, and inducing a calming (mild sedative) effect.

A few scientific studies have been conducted to test specific effects resulting from schisandra supplementation. In one study, patients with a certain heart malady (dilated cardiomyopathy) were given a combination of panax ginseng, radix ophiopogonis, and schisandra. The subjects' improvement was measured via an echocardiogram as well as a treadmill tolerance test. After taking the herbal blend for forty days, heart function improved significantly and exercise tolerance increased by more than 67 percent. Studies of exercise have shown schisandra to increase work capacity (in running mice) and lessen the rise in cortisol in athletes undergoing heavy training.

Schisandra is generally considered to be safe and nontoxic when used as directed. Typical dosage recommendations are in the range of 100–500 mg per day. Commercial schisandra supplements may be found as stand-alone products or as blends with multiple ingredients (such as ginseng and rhodiola) targeting energy and performance. Reported side effects resulting from schisandra ingestion include mild indigestion and skin rash. Because schisandra may induce uterine muscle contractions (similar to the effects of ashwagandha), pregnant women should not take the herb.

RHODIOLA

Rhodiola (*Rhodiola rosea/Rhodiola crenulata*) comprises several species of plants from the Arctic mountain regions of Siberia. The root of the plant is used medicinally and is also known as *Arctic root* or *golden root* and more recently as *crenulin*. Rhodiola has been used for centuries to treat cold and flulike symptoms, promote longevity, and increase the body's resistance to physical and mental stresses. It is typically considered to be an adaptogen (like ginseng) and is believed to invigorate the body and mind to increase resistance to a multitude of stresses. The key active constituents in rhodiola are believed to be rosavin, rosarin, rosin, and salidroside.

In one open clinical trial, rhodiola rosea extract was effective in reducing or removing symptoms of depression in 65 percent of the patients studied. In another open-label study, twenty-six out of thirty-five men suffering from weak erections or premature ejaculation reported improvements in sexual function following treatment with 100–150 mg of rhodiola rosea extract for three months. In another study, of physicians during nighttime hospital duty, 175 mg per day of rhodiola (standardized to 4.5 mg salidroside) for two weeks resulted in a significant improvement in associative thinking, short-term memory, concentration, and speed of audiovisual perception. An additional study of students undergoing a stressful twenty-day period of exams showed that 50 mg per day of rhodiola alleviated mental fatigue and improved well-being.

Overall, rhodiola rosea extract appears to be valuable as an adaptogen, specifically in increasing the body's ability to deal with a number of psychological and physiological stresses. Of particular value is the theoretical role for rhodiola in increasing the body's ability to take up and utilize oxygen—an effect similar to that of cordyceps (see Chapter 11)—which may explain some of the non-stimulant "energizing" effects attributed to the plant. Rhodiola is often called the poor-man's cordyceps because of ancient stories in which Chinese commoners used rhodiola for energy because the plants grew wild throughout the countryside, while only the emperor and his immediate family and concubines were allowed access to the rare cordyceps mushroom.

Rhodiola rosea extract is thought to be quite safe. There are no known contraindications or interactions with other drugs or herbs, but potential exists for mild allergic reactions (rashes) in some individuals. General dosage recommendations for rhodiola rosea extract are typically in the range of 100–300 mg per day. Like schisandra, rhodiola can be purchased either as a stand-alone product or in combination with other ingredients.

ASTRAGALUS

Astragalus is an herb recommended as much for stimulation of the immune system as for its energy-promoting properties. Perhaps because chronic stress can deplete both energy levels and increase the risk of illness and infection, astragalus may be particularly beneficial in individuals who feel fatigued due to high levels of emotional and physical stress. Athletes in particular may benefit from astragalus supplementation because intense training and competition are often associated with an increased incidence of colds and other upper respiratory tract infections, conditions for which astragalus is thought to be most effective.

Astragalus has been used as an herbal tonic for centuries in traditional Chinese medicine (TCM) and in Native American folk medicine. As a tonic, astragalus is used primarily as a "prevention" herb throughout the cold and flu season—a different usage from the more popular echinacea (Chapter 11), which is best used for early-stage treatment as soon as you feel a cold or the flu coming on. In TCM, astragalus is often combined with other tonic herbs, such as ginseng, cordyceps, or ashwagandha, to keep the immune system humming during periods of high stress.

There have been some clinical tests of astragalus on humans, most of which come from China, where the herb appears to stimulate the immune system in patients with infections. At least one clinical trial in the U.S. has shown astragalus to boost levels of T cells (a type of infection-fighting white blood cell) to near-normal ranges in some cancer patients, suggesting the possibility of a synergistic effect of astragalus with chemotherapy. Most of what we know about astragalus, however, comes from test-tube and animal experiments, which show that it can help fight bacteria and viruses by enhancing various aspects of the body's normal immune response; specifically, it enhances function of specific immune-system cells such as T cells, lymphocytes, and neutrophils. In animal studies, astragalus extracts are effective in preventing infection of mice by the influenza virus, possibly by increasing the phagocytotic activity of the white blood cells of the immune system.

When used as recommended, astragalus has no known side effects, at high intakes gastrointestinal distress and diarrhea are possible. Although astragalus is available as a single-ingredient supplement (250–500 mg per day), it may be even more effective in lower doses (100–200 mg per day) when combined with other immune-stimulating herbs and nutrients.

Summary

As part of the hierarchy of natural cortisol-controlling compounds, adaptogens certainly represent a powerful and effective solution for counteracting many of the detrimental effects of stress. Within that hierarchy, however, the adaptogenic herbs are probably best thought of as temporary or occasional-use agents during periods of particularly high stress.

In this context:

- A solid foundation of multivitamin and multimineral supplementation is the first step in a good plan for fighting stress (featuring vitamin C, magnesium, etc., as detailed in Chapter 7);

- The next step should be targeted cortisol-modulating supplements (including theanine, epimedium, etc., as outlined in Chapter 8);

- And then should come the reinforcements against episodes of stress in the form of a balanced adaptogen regimen, as covered in this chapter.

. . . .
. . .
. . .
. . .
                      :

CHAPTER 10

Relaxation and
Calming Supplements

Ⅰt is no surprise that dietary supplements marketed for promoting relaxation, reducing anxiety, and alleviating stress are among the top-selling products on the market. Millions of tired and stressed-out people (many of whom may be reading this book) can relate to promises of natural products that will enhance their brain function and make them feel better.

As discussed previously, physiologists and nutritionists regularly document the dramatic improvements in mood, emotions, confidence, and self-efficacy that result from some very simple lifestyle modifications. Regular exercise and adequate diet can result in profound changes in the body's own production of mood-elevating chemicals, such as the endorphins that cause "runner's high" and the neurotransmitters like serotonin that contribute to emotional well-being. In general terms, *any amount* of exercise can help to induce feelings of relaxation and calmness. Walking for twenty minutes on as many days of the week as possible (but at least three times per week) might be a good place to start.

On the nutritional side of things, it will probably come as no surprise that diet is intimately tied to emotions. Just think about your feelings as you contemplate gorging yourself on that hot fudge sundae (weakness), followed by your feelings when you finally give in to the temptation (guilt) and start eating (elation), until you get to the bottom of the bowl (disappointment). All kidding aside, the foods we eat *directly* influence our moods, because the macronutrients (carbohydrates, proteins, fats) and micronutrients (vitamins, minerals, and phytonutrients) they contain ultimately act as potent neurochemicals. For example, a higher-protein diet can leave some people feeling energized, while a higher-carbohydrate diet can leave others feeling hungry, lethargic, and depressed.

For most people, the best advice for getting a handle on their emotional balance is to take a week or so to analyze how their diet affects their mood. Pay attention to every speck of food you eat and how it makes you feel. This is made easier by keeping a "food and mood" diary for seven to ten days, wherein you record every bite of food eaten, time of day eaten, and mood and energy levels before and afterward. The patterns revealed in a food diary can be enlightening. But if the thought of adding such a task to your busy schedule stresses you out, then a less formal period of observation can be informative, too. Once you feel you know a bit about how certain foods influence your emotions, then you can decide where some of the dietary supplements outlined below may (or may not) fit into your lifestyle.

In very general terms, a number of popular herbs are used to help "take the edge off" after a particularly stressful day. Many of the herbs in this category are found in relaxing herbal teas and include chamomile, melissa, lemon balm, hops, oats, skullcap, and passionflower. Even though these herbs are widely used to help soothe ragged nerves (again, mostly as herbal teas), none of them have any strong or convincing scientific evidence to support their effectiveness against stress, anxiety, or elevated cortisol levels. That certainly doesn't mean they are useless—after all, a warm cup of tea can sometimes be just the thing to help reduce stress and bring you back to a more relaxed state.

Some of the more specific and effective dietary supplements for promoting relaxation include those listed in Table 10.1, and they are outlined in greater detail in the rest of the chapter. Many of these supplements are also used to treat mild forms of depression, anxiety, and insomnia, but they all have a general calming quality that can contribute to overall feelings of relaxation.

Table 10.1: Popular Antistress Supplements Frequently Used to Treat Depression, Anxiety, and Insomnia

Supplement	Dose (per Day)	Primary Effect
Kava kava	50–150 mg	Antianxiety
Melatonin	1–10 mg	Antianxiety/sleep aid
Valerian	250–500 mg	Antianxiety/sleep aid
Gotu kola	60–180 mg	Antianxiety
St. John's wort	450–900 mg	Relieves mild depression
5-HTP	300–900 mg	Relieves mild depression
DLPA	75–200 mg	Elevates mood
SAM-e	200–600 mg	Relieves mild depression

KAVA KAVA

Kava (*Piper methysticum*) is a root from a pepper plant used for centuries by Pacific Islanders (e.g., Fijians and Hawaiians) as a ceremonial intoxicant to help people relax and socialize. Modern-day usage of kava is as a dietary supplement for relieving anxiety and tension. The active ingredients in kava, chemicals called *kavalactones*, act as a mild central-nervous-system depressant, but typically do not produce the hangover effects associated with alcohol.

Traditional preparation of the kava root involves cutting up freshly dug roots, chewing them, and then spitting them into a large communal bowl containing water or coconut milk. This unappetizing combination is then mixed, strained to remove any remaining large pieces, and passed around for everyone to share. It all sounds (and tastes!) pretty disgusting, but early Christian missionaries to the islands actually tried to ban kava parties because people were having such a good time preparing and passing the kava drinks. If you can't stomach the chewing and spitting part of kava preparation, the roots can be pounded until soft, then soaked in a fluid before drinking. The brew has a somewhat bitter taste and a slightly numbing or tingling sensation on the tongue.

Of course, kava is not very often prepared or consumed in the traditional way by average supplement users in the United States. Instead, the kava roots are dried and ground into a powder by machines. The powder can then be packed into capsules or tablets, blended into drinks, or dissolved in an alcohol-based extract. Americans spend about $30–$50 million annually on kava-containing products—a powerful testament to our high-stress lifestyles and our need for help in relaxing.

Although few well-designed studies have been conducted in the United States on kava in humans, several projects have been carried out in Europe. These trials have mostly been conducted in Germany, and have found kava (at a dose containing 50–150 mg per day of kavalactones) to be helpful in alleviating anxiety and other emotional problems related to stress. One study assessed various psychological stressors, and found that after four weeks the group taking kava supplements showed significant decreases in stress in every category measured, in contrast to the placebo group, which showed little variation in any area.

No side effects or withdrawal symptoms have been noted during kava-supplementation studies or when people stopped taking the supplement, but recently several case studies have shown that kava supplementation may be linked to various forms of liver damage in some people. In light of these findings, some supplement companies are voluntarily removing their kava-containing products from the market. Additionally, the U.S. Food and Drug Administration in early 2002 issued a warning that kava carries a "potential risk" of causing severe liver damage and urging kava users and their doctors to be on the lookout for signs of liver injury. Therefore, until we know more about the potential liver toxicity associated with kava supplements, it would be prudent for people with liver damage to avoid kava and for healthy people to consume no more than 50 mg of kavalactones per day.

Because kava depresses the nervous system, it should not be taken with alcohol or in conjunction with antianxiety drugs. In addition, although kava appears to be helpful for alleviating cases of mild to moderate anxiety, self-medication with kava is probably not appropriate for individuals with major anxiety conditions. It is also advisable to refrain from using kava before driving. An interesting case occurred in Maryland a few years ago wherein a police officer pulled over a man for driving erratically. The man slurred his speech and had difficulty walking, so the officer assumed he was intoxicated, despite the man's insistence that he had not been drinking. Blood-alcohol measures indicated no alcohol in the man's system. After further questioning, it was discovered that the man had recently consumed several cups of kava tea.

MELATONIN

Melatonin is a hormone produced in the pineal gland of the brain from the amino acid tryptophan. It is used in the body to help regulate sleep/wake cycles. Melatonin levels are lowest during midday and highest at night. Daylight is known to slow the production of melatonin, while darkness increases its production.

Dietary supplements containing melatonin promote relaxation and sleep, but the best evidence of its effectiveness comes from studies of people who have disturbed sleep/wake cycles, such as from jet lag and shift work. Several studies show that low-dose melatonin supplements (1–5 mg taken thirty to sixty minutes before bedtime) can help people sleep better, fall asleep faster, and have higher energy and alertness levels upon waking. Theoretical reasons also exist for melatonin's offering benefits in alleviating depression, especially the type of depression brought on by a lack of sunlight during winter months and often referred to as *seasonal affective disorder* (SAD, also known as the "winter blues"). On the other hand, some studies suggest that melatonin can induce or deepen depression in susceptible individuals.

The interaction of melatonin with other supplements or drugs is unknown, but melatonin supplements may be dangerous for people with cardiovascular risks, due to the possibility of vasoconstriction and increased blood pressure. Additionally, the National Institutes of Health have warned about possible dangers of melatonin supplementation, including infertility, reduced sex drive in males, hypothermia, retinal damage, and interference with hormone replacement therapy. Information regarding the long-term effects of melatonin supplements is unavailable.

Melatonin can be viewed as a relatively inexpensive and non-addictive alternative to over-the-counter chemical sleep aids. It may be particularly useful as a short-term regulator of sleep/wake cycles in cases such as getting the body clock back on schedule after crossing several time zones (jet lag). Studies of melatonin as a sleep aid or for relief of symptoms associated with jet lag have shown 1–10 mg to be effective, depending on the degree of sleep disturbance. Be careful, though, because the higher end of this dosage range can cause some people to experience vivid nightmares. High-dose melatonin supplements (around 50 mg) may disrupt female fertility and menstrual patterns and should be avoided except under the supervision of a reproductive physician.

VALERIAN

Valerian (*Valeriana officinalis*) has been used as a medicinal antianxiety herb and sleep aid since the days of the Romans. The dried roots of the plant are used in teas, tinctures, capsules, and tablets for promoting relaxation, inducing sleep, calming nerves, and reducing anxiety. It is unclear which of valerian's numerous compounds is the true active ingredient, but the combination of compounds appears to work together in the brain in a manner similar to the action of prescription tranquilizers such as Valium and Halcion. One problem, however, is that valerian is notoriously unstable; it loses its activity very quickly if it is not processed, packaged, and stored in exactly the right way.

Numerous studies in animals and humans support the effect of valerian as a mild sedative and sleep aid. In several studies, 400–600 mg of valerian extract, taken approximately one hour before bedtime, provides benefits in terms of overall relaxation, reduction of tension, and ability to fall asleep. Some products combine valerian with support herbs such as hops or melissa (lemon balm), both of which offer additional relaxation benefits of their own with none of valerian's characteristic sweaty-sock odor.

Taken before bedtime, valerian appears to reduce the amount of time required to fall asleep. It is unknown, however, whether the quality of the sleep is affected by valerian consumption. Valerian is generally regarded as a mild tranquilizer and has been deemed safe by the German Commission E (the German regulatory body for herbal medicines) for treating "restlessness and sleeping disorders brought on by nervous conditions."

Because the activity and strength of valerian preparations can vary significantly from one product to the next, it is recommended whenever possible to select a standardized preparation containing 0.5–1.0 percent valerenic acids and to follow the package instructions on the particular product. As a general guideline, approximately 250–500 mg of a 5-to-1 or 6-to-1 extract can be taken before bed (as a sleep aid) or as needed as a mild tranquilizer.

Although valerian does not appear to be habit-forming or to result in hangover-like morning drowsiness, it does seem to impair one's ability to concentrate for a few hours after taking it. Occasional reports of headaches and mild nausea are documented, but habituation or dependency is unlikely when it is used as directed. Valerian should be avoided by pregnant and lactating women, and by children. Individuals currently taking sedative drugs or antidepressant medications should consult with their personal physician before taking valerian, and no one should take the herb in conjunction with alcohol or other tranquilizers, or for more than two weeks.

> *Mark,* the building contractor whom we met in Chapter 4, struggled with stress-related insomnia. Mark already got a great deal of physical activity at work, and because his wife (a fitness instructor) knew a lot about nutrition, he had help in eating a very well balanced diet. He started on a supplement regimen that was targeted to control his cortisol levels and help him relax and sleep better. Mark's program included both theanine (100 mg taken with a bottle of water as he left the job site in the late afternoon) and valerian (250 mg taken thirty minutes before bedtime). The theanine helped him to relax without getting drowsy on his way home from work, and the valerian helped him to relax just a bit more and drop off to sleep faster. (For more about theanine, see Chapter 8.) After only a few days on this regimen, Mark reported a deeper and more restful sleep than he had experienced in months. As a result of his better sleep quality, Mark's energy levels went up and his ability to concentrate at work was much improved.

GOTU KOLA

Gotu kola (*Centella asiatica*) is an Indian herb that has been used for centuries in Ayurvedic (Indian) and traditional Chinese medicine to alleviate symptoms of depression and anxiety. Several animal studies have shown that gotu kola enhances performance in maze tests (which assess memory and learning ability as well as anxiety) and reduces various symptoms of stress. Findings from human studies also suggest a beneficial effect of gotu kola in reducing anxiety and responses to laboratory-induced stress. It is interesting to note that a number of laboratory studies have also shown gotu kola to bind to specialized cellular receptors in the gastrointestinal tract called cholecystokinin (CCK) receptors. CCK receptors help regulate appetite, food intake, and eating behavior, and the binding of gotu kola to them may help modulate hunger and food cravings throughout the day, especially those cravings and urges for bingeing that can be brought on by stress. It is important to keep in mind that gotu kola should not be confused with the kola nut, which is completely unrelated and is often used in weight-loss and energy supplements as a natural source of caffeine.

In one investigation of the anxiolytic (antianxiety) effects of gotu kola, twenty healthy volunteers were given either a single 12-gram dose of gotu kola or a look-alike placebo. Results showed that compared with placebo, gotu kola significantly reduced the response of the subjects to a series of laboratory stressors (loud noises and other startling events) administered over the next thirty to sixty minutes. Now, 12 grams is a pretty large dose of gotu kola, but the effect was quite fast and very powerful. Smaller doses are known to be effective in reducing stress response during normal, everyday stressors of the sort that most of us would encounter on a regular basis.

The activity of gotu kola has also been studied in another form of stress: that of injury. In animal studies, gotu kola extracts have been shown to increase the production of hydroxyproline and collagen, the structural components needed for wound healing, by 50–60 percent. Other studies have shown gotu kola to possess antioxidant effects that can be beneficial in wound healing, skin protection, and immune-system support. In these studies, the antioxidant effects of gotu kola, given twice daily for seven days, improved antioxidant capacity of the tissue by 35–75 percent and reduced free-radical damage by nearly 70 percent.

Gotu kola is frequently found in topical skin preparations for its benefits in speeding wound healing; dietary forms of the herb are generally provided in capsule or tablet form. Dietary intake of gotu kola appears to be nontoxic, but there is some anecdotal evidence that gotu kola may result in elevated blood-sugar levels, an effect that could be of concern to individuals with diabetes. Typical dosage recommendations are in the range of 60–180 mg per day of an extract standardized to contain 30–40 percent of the active triterpene compounds (asiaticoside, asiatic acid, and related compounds).

ST. JOHN'S WORT

St. John's wort (*Hypericum perforatum*) is typically recommended as an herbal alternative to antidepressant medications. It is effective in balancing mood and lifting spirits, and in many people it is also quite beneficial in relieving the fatigue that is often associated with mild to moderate depression and high stress. People who are depressed or under constant stress often lack the energy to even get themselves out of bed in the morning, and their day is a never-ending battle against fatigue. By correcting neurotransmitter imbalances in the brain, St. John's wort can bring energy levels back to normal and help alleviate the crushing fatigue that accompanies depressed mood and chronic stress.

The precise active ingredients in St. John's wort are unknown, but extracts standardized to contain 0.3 percent hypericin and 3 percent hyperforin, in doses of 900 mg per day, are known to be effective in alleviating mild to moderate depressive symptoms. St. John's wort is readily available as capsules containing the standardized extract. Using these hypericin/hyperforin extracts, numerous clinical studies have shown that people with mild or moderate depression tend to respond to St. John's wort to about the same degree as they would to some of the older prescription antidepressant medications, with fewer side effects. A number of well-controlled studies comparing the St. John's wort extract to prescription antidepressants such as fluoxetine (Prozac), sertraline (Zoloft), and paroxetine (Paxil) have found St. John's wort to be comparable in effectiveness, but superior to prescription drugs with regard to tolerability. Overall, more than a dozen double-blind placebo-controlled studies have been conducted—albeit mostly small studies—and the majority support the case for the effectiveness of St. John's wort in alleviating mild to moderate depression, but not severe depression.

St. John's wort is quite safe in terms of observed side effects, the most common of which are mild gastrointestinal upset, mild allergic reactions (skin rash), and insomnia/restlessness, usually when taken close to bedtime. There have been no published reports of serious adverse side effects from taking the herb alone, and animal studies using large doses of St. John's wort have not shown any serious problems. The most commonly studied adverse effect of St. John's wort is its ability to cause photosensitivity in fair-skinned individuals, increasing their risk of sunburn.

Although direct side effects from consuming St. John's wort appear to be quite rare, several recent reports have raised the possibility that the herb may interact with and decrease the effectiveness of various medications, including HIV drugs (protease inhibitors), immunosuppressants (such as cyclosporin for organ transplants), digoxin (for congestive heart failure), blood thinners (Coumadin/warfarin), chemotherapy drugs (olanzapine/clozapine), and asthma medications (theophylline). If you are currently taking any of these, or other prescription medications, *discontinue* taking *or do not begin* taking St. John's wort without first consulting your personal physician (abrupt withdrawal of the herb could increase blood levels of various medications, which could be dangerous in certain cases).

St. John's wort appears to be helpful in about 50 to 60 percent of cases, but as with prescription antidepressants the full effect takes about four to six weeks to develop. It is important to note that St. John's wort should *never* be used for the treatment of severe depression (feelings of suicide, extreme inability to cope with daily life, severe anxiety, or extreme fatigue); in such cases, physician-directed drug therapy may mean the difference between life and death.

5-HTP

5-HTP (5-hydroxytryptophan) is a derivative of the amino acid tryptophan. In the body, tryptophan is converted into 5-HTP, which can then be converted into serotonin, a potent neurotransmitter in the brain. Although 5-HTP is not found at any significant level in a normal diet, tryptophan is found in a wide variety of protein foods. The 5-HTP used in dietary supplements is derived from the seeds of an African plant, *Griffonia simplicifolia*, and is typically used as a treatment for relieving mild depression, counteracting insomnia, promoting weight loss, and reducing overall sensations of stress and pain such as migraine headaches, fibromyalgia, and general muscle pain.

5-HTP is typically used to treat mild depression and combat stress based on the theory that as a precursor to serotonin, supplements of 5-HTP can increase serotonin levels and influence mood, sleep patterns, and pain control. In a few small studies, 5-HTP has been shown to be as effective as prescription antidepressant medications—and with fewer side effects. In other studies, doses of 5-HTP in the range of 300–900 mg per day have resulted in benefits in reducing pain associated with migraines and fibromyalgia, reducing appetite, and promoting sleep, possibly by increasing blood levels of melatonin. It appears that there are "responders," individuals who experience an elevation in 5-HTP levels in the blood, as well as "nonresponders," who see no such increase.

The most significant safety concern related to 5-HTP supplements is the remote possibility for contamination with a compound linked to a disorder known as *eosinophilic myalgia syndrome* (EMS), which results in muscle pain and weakness, vomiting, headache, and, in rare cases, death. In 1989 an outbreak of EMS was linked to contaminated tryptophan supplements—not to the tryptophan per se, but to a contaminant in the supplements. As a result, the FDA banned the sale of all tryptophan supplements, a move that has been widely criticized by people on both sides of the supplement debate. The banned tryptophan supplements were manufactured from a bacterial source in a fermentation process, whereas 5-HTP is extracted from the seeds of a plant—so it is less likely (though not impossible) that the contaminant associated with EMS, commonly known as *peak* X, is present in 5-HTP supplements. Some supplement manufacturers and raw-material suppliers conduct quality-control tests to confirm the absence of peak X in their 5-HTP supplements. If you decide to try 5-HTP, it is suggested that you contact the manufacturer of your supplement for confirmation that their products have passed this type of analysis. Supplemental forms of 5-HTP are available in capsule or tablet form, as extracts from griffonia seeds (providing 15–20 percent 5-HTP), and in synthetic form (99 percent pure).

In addition to the above safety considerations, 5-HTP supplements are not recommended for children or for women who are pregnant or lactating. People currently taking prescription antidepressants, weight-control medications, or herbal remedies for depression (such as St. John's wort) should not combine these treatments with 5-HTP supplements, except on the advice and guidance of a nutritionally oriented physician.

D, L-PHENYLALANINE (DLPA)

Phenylalanine is an essential amino acid, meaning that the body cannot synthesize it on its own and therefore a person must get it from her or his diet. The primary dietary sources of phenylalanine are high-protein foods such as meat, fish, eggs, and dairy products. Another significant dietary source for some people may be sugar-free products containing the artificial sweetener aspartame (Nutrasweet), which is formed by a combination of phenylalanine with another amino acid, aspartic acid.

Amino acids exist in two forms, designated as "L" and "D" forms. The L form is the naturally occurring form in foods, whereas the D form is the synthetic variety. When an amino acid is synthesized commercially, there is usually a mixture of the L and D forms. Sometimes the D form is removed, but in the case of phenylalanine, the combination of the two forms is used to take advantage of the unique characteristics of each form. The combined form of the supplement is known as D, L-phenylalanine, or DLPA, and is typically used for relieving depression, combating stress, elevating mood, decreasing pain, boosting memory, and suppressing appetite.

DLPA has two distinct fates in the body. The L form of phenylalanine can be converted in the body to another amino acid, tyrosine. Tyrosine, as we already learned in Chapter 8, can be converted into one of several neurotransmitter molecules—dopamine, norepinephrine, and epinephrine—each of which has important functions in brain metabolism and the general stress response. The D form of phenylalanine *cannot* be converted to tyrosine, but it can be converted to another compound called *phenylethylamine*, which may have effects in elevating mood, treating depression, and altering pain sensation.

DLPA has been used to treat depression, Parkinson's disease, and painful conditions such as arthritis and fibromyalgia. In one study, phenylalanine supplements were able to elevate mood in thirty-one of forty subjects suffering from depression. Doses of DLPA from 75–200 mg per day over twenty days have been shown to be effective in treating depressed mood, agitation, anxiety, and sleep disturbances.

Like 5-HTP, DLPA may have some benefits for people who are concerned with possible drug/herb interactions reported for St. John's wort. Rarely used as a stand-alone supplement, DLPA may be better suited as an ingredient in a larger blend of nutrients and herbs targeting pain and depression, stress and anxiety, and appetite and weight loss. The daily requirement of phenylalanine is probably about 1 gram, easily obtained in the diet. Effective DLPA doses are in the range of 75–200 mg per day. This dose of DLPA appears low when viewed in light of the 1 gram of dietary phenylalanine recommended. The difference is that the dietary phenylalanine (all L form) can be converted into tyrosine (a good thing) but not into phenylethylamine (the painkilling antidepressant stuff), because that only comes from the D form of phenylalanine. Because DLPA is 50 percent D-phenylalanine, the supplement provides a raw material for conversion into phenylethylamine that is not provided in the diet.

SAM-E

S-adenosylmethionine (SAM-e) is a form of the sulfur-containing amino acid methionine, combined with adenosine (part of the energy compound ATP). Like methionine, SAM-e is involved in numerous metabolic processes in the body that require sulfur— such as the methylation reactions. The body typically manufactures all the SAM-e it requires from methionine consumed in protein foods, but a defect in methylation or a deficiency in any of the cofactors required for SAM-e production (such as methionine, choline, or the B vitamins) is theorized to reduce the body's ability to produce SAM-e.

It has been hypothesized that a defect in the body's methylation process is central to the biochemical basis of certain neuropsychiatric disorders, and that chronic stress can interfere with the body's ability to conduct these methylation reactions. Tissue levels of SAM-e have been found to be low in the elderly and in patients suffering from depression and chronic stress. SAM-e has performed as well as conventional antidepressant drugs in studies of depression, probably due to an increase in brain levels of neurotransmitters such as serotonin and dopamine.

SAM-e is quite safe at recommended doses and has the distinct advantage over some other herbal medicines of being a naturally occurring compound in the body, which suggests that supplementation with SAM-e simply provides an additional dietary source of this nutrient. Other antidepressant compounds that are available as dietary supplements, such as St. John's wort, could be viewed as more of a pharmacological approach to relieving depression because they are not naturally found in the body. The problem with dietary supplements containing SAM-e is their cost— SAM-e is not an inexpensive ingredient. The good news, however, is that the mood benefits of SAM-e are more affordable (delivered at 200–600 mg per day) than the joint-health benefits of the supplement (for which you'd need 1,200–1,400 mg per day). Even at 200–600 mg per day, however, SAM-e tablets (the most stable form) generally cost $20 to $30 for a ten-day supply.

──────────── Summary ────────────

So where do these calming herbs fit in? They can certainly represent an effective approach to promoting relaxation and destressing a person during periods of particularly high stress. However, when it comes to designing your specific cortisol-control regimen, it may be helpful to take it step-by-step (see sidebar). As such, most of the supplements covered in this chapter should be thought of as secondary choices to be used in specific cases of depression, insomnia, or when something is needed to take the edge off after a particularly stressful day.

We've now covered the five most important steps for controlling stress and modulating cortisol levels with supplements:

1. Avoid excessive doses of supplements that can increase cortisol levels (herbal stimulants such as ephedra, covered in Chapter 6)
2. Take a multivitamin/multimineral supplement as a cortisol-control foundation (covered in Chapter 7)
3. Focus on targeted cortisol-modulating supplements, especially during periods of high stress (covered in Chapter 8)
4. Consider adding "reinforcement" supplements against stress in the form of adaptogens (covered in Chapter 9)
5. Use calming supplements to fight depression, insomnia, and frazzled nerves (covered in Chapter 10)

Stressed Jess will have to follow each of these five steps for optimal cortisol control, with particular emphasis on step 3.

Strained Jane may be able to get away with following only steps 1–3; she may never have a need to progress to steps 4 and 5.

Relaxed Jack, as laid back as he appears, can also benefit from following the first two steps on a regular basis, but he may need to progress to step 3 during his occasional high-stress periods.

CHAPTER 11

Metabolic-Support Supplements (Blood-Sugar Control, Muscle Maintenance, and Immune Enhancement)

I f you're following each of the five most important steps listed in the sidebar at the end of Chapter 10, then you're doing just about all you can do with dietary supplements to control stress and modulate cortisol levels. In certain cases, however, there may be reason to specifically address some of the detrimental effects of chronically elevated cortisol—namely, its effects on blood sugar, muscle loss, and immune suppression. In each of these cases, a handful of supplements exists that can have a beneficial effect; these are not necessarily supplements that need to be used on a regular basis, as one should use multivitamin/mineral and cortisol-controlling supplements.

BLOOD-SUGAR CONTROL

Before you say "ho-hum" to the idea of blood-sugar control, remember from Chapter 4 that optimal control of blood sugar is closely related to prevention of diabetes, heart disease, syndrome X, appetite

control, and obesity. If any of these chronic conditions are of importance to you (and they should be), then so too is blood-sugar control.

Luckily, many of our blood-sugar-control needs will be
addressed by our comprehensive multivitamin/multimineral foundation—provided that it contains chromium, vanadium, vitamin
E, and a blend of B-complex vitamins and antioxidants. Of primary importance for blood-sugar control are the trace minerals
chromium and vanadium, both of which are involved in the
actions of insulin in regulating blood-sugar levels. And for people
who need additional blood-sugar control, two powerful Indian
herbs can help keep blood sugar from rising too high or falling too
low: banaba and gymnema.

Chromium

Chromium is an essential trace mineral that aids in glucose
metabolism, insulin regulation, appetite control, and cholesterol
maintenance. Chromium deficiency is known to lead to glucose
intolerance and insulin resistance, symptoms commonly encountered in people with diabetes. Since chromium helps regulate the
actions of insulin (as a constituent of glucose tolerance factor),
chromium supplements may help support the many functions of
insulin in the body, such as maintaining blood sugar and cholesterol levels and controlling appetite (particularly sweet cravings).
In diabetic and overweight individuals, chromium supplements
have been shown to reduce triglyceride levels, improve glucose
tolerance, and normalize insulin levels. Supplements of 400 mcg
(micrograms) have helped overweight women lose about 50 percent more fat in three months compared to a placebo group,
probably due to a direct effect on controlling blood-sugar levels
and modulating appetite and cravings.

Chromium is one of the most widely available trace minerals;
a good multivitamin/mineral supplement should provide 200 mcg.
Specialized blood-sugar-control supplements often provide
another 200–400 mcg of chromium in a blend of related ingredients such as vanadium, banaba, and gymnema.

Vanadium

Vanadium is another trace element that promotes normal insulin function. Safe and adequate dietary intakes fall within the range of approximately 10–100 mcg per day. Vanadium is thought to mimic the physiological effects of insulin by a mechanism that remains unclear. Through this insulin-mimetic effect, vanadium is thought to promote glycogen synthesis, maintain blood-glucose levels, and stimulate protein synthesis for muscle growth. Vanadyl sulfate supplements have been shown to normalize blood-glucose levels and reduce glycosylated hemoglobin levels in patients with diabetes.

A balanced multivitamin/mineral supplement may provide 10 mcg of vanadium—but check the label, because many multis contain no vanadium at all. Specialized supplements for blood-sugar control may provide another 30–60 mcg of vanadium, but there is no need for your daily intake of vanadium to exceed 100 mcg. At the recommended doses (10–100 mcg per day), vanadium is considered quite safe, but some bodybuilding supplements are known to contain vanadium at milligram levels—about one thousand times higher than the amounts needed for blood-sugar control, and probably associated with long-term damage to the liver and kidneys.

Banaba

Banaba leaf (*Lagestroemia speciosa*) is a medicinal plant that grows in India, Southeast Asia, and the Philippines. Traditional uses include brewing tea from the leaves as a treatment for diabetes and hyperglycemia (elevated blood sugar). The hypoglycemic (blood-sugar-lowering) effect of banaba leaf extract is similar to that of insulin, which induces glucose transport from the blood into body cells. The blood-sugar-regulating properties of banaba in both animals and humans have been demonstrated in studies of isolated cells. In isolated cells, the active ingredient in banaba extract, corosolic acid, is known to stimulate glucose uptake. In diabetic mice, rats, and rabbits, banaba feeding reduces elevated blood sugar and insulin levels to normal. In humans with type-2 diabetes, banaba extract, at a dose of 16–48 mg per day for four to eight weeks, has been shown to be effective in reducing blood-sugar levels (5–30 percent reduction) and maintaining tighter control of blood-sugar fluctuations. An interesting side effect of tighter control of blood sugar and insulin levels is a tendency of banaba to promote weight loss—at an average of two to four pounds per month—without significant dietary alterations. It is likely that modulation of glucose and insulin levels reduces total caloric intake somewhat and encourages moderate weight loss.

Commercial preparations of banaba leaf extract are available in powder, tablet, or capsule forms from a number of manufacturers. Banaba may be most effective when it is combined with chromium and vanadium in products to control blood sugar and appetite, and to promote weight loss.

> Remember *Paul,* the lawyer from Chapter 4 whose weight went up as his responsibilities (and, not coincidentally, his stress levels) increased? Paul was a perfect example of a person who was doing many things "right" in terms of his diet and exercise patterns, but his efforts were being hampered or blocked by his high-stress lifestyle and his elevated cortisol levels. By continuing his balanced approach to diet and exercise, Paul had already been keeping his cortisol levels from shooting sky high, but he was finally able to solve his weight issues by adding targeted dietary supplementation.
>
> For Paul, the supplements of choice were theanine (50 mg in the A.M. and 100 mg in the P.M.) and banaba (16 mg with each meal). He decided on these herbs because of theanine's dual benefits in promoting relaxation and improving mental focus (both of which could benefit Paul as a lawyer), and for the effects of banaba in helping to regulate blood-sugar levels and control appetite. (For more about theanine, see Chapter 8.) Within a few days of starting this supplementation plan, Paul noticed that he was experiencing more restful sleep at night, enhanced energy and mental focus during the day, and an extreme reduction in his cravings for those "bad" foods when his workload went up. Over a period of six weeks—and largely due to improvements in sleep quality, cortisol control, and appetite regulation—Paul was able

to drop eight pounds of body weight and fit into business suits
he had been unable to wear for more than a year.

Gymnema

Gymnema (*Gymnema sylvestre*) is a plant used medicinally in India
and Southeast Asia for treatment of "sweet urine," or what we
refer to in the West as diabetes or hyperglycemia (high blood
sugar). In ancient Indian texts, gymnema is referred to as *gurmar*,
which means "sugar destroyer" in Sanskrit. Gymnema leaves,
whether extracted or infused into a tea, suppress glucose absorption and reduce the sensation of sweetness in foods—effects that
may deliver important health benefits for individuals who want to
reduce blood-sugar levels or body weight. The hypoglycemic
(blood-sugar-lowering) effect of gymnema has been known for centuries, and modern scientific methods have isolated at least nine
different fractions of gymnemic acids that possess hypoglycemic
activity. Very high doses of dried gymnema leaves may even help to
repair the cellular damage that causes diabetes by helping to regen-
erate the insulin-producing beta cells in the pancreas. Several
human studies conducted on gymnema for treatment of type-2 diabetes have shown significant reduction in blood glucose, glycosylated hemoglobin (an index of blood-sugar control), and insulin
requirements, allowing insulin therapy to be reduced.

Gymnema appears to increase the effectiveness of insulin
rather than causing the body to produce more, although the precise mechanism by which this occurs remains unknown. The
effect of gymnema extract on lowering blood levels of glucose,
cholesterol, and triglycerides is fairly gradual, typically taking a
few days to several weeks. As with other natural ingredients for
control of blood sugar and insulin levels, such as banaba leaf
extract, a common side effect is weight loss, probably due to a
combination of appetite suppression and control of food cravings,
especially for carbohydrates and sweets.

As with banaba, supplements containing gymnema often combine the herb into capsules with chromium and/or vanadium for

optimal effectiveness. At typical recommended doses (200–400 mg per day), dietary supplements containing gymnema are not associated with significant adverse side effects. A person may experience mild gastrointestinal upset if he or she takes gymnema on an empty stomach, so consumption of the supplement with meals is recommended. Caution is urged, however, with extremely high doses, which may have the potential to induce hypoglycemia (abnormally low blood sugar) in susceptible individuals. People with active diabetes should consult their personal physician before and during use of gymnema, as alterations to their dosage of insulin or other antidiabetic medications may be warranted. Certain medications, including the antidepressant St. John's wort as well as the salicylates (aspirin and white willow bark), can enhance the blood-sugar-lowering effects of gymnema, whereas certain stimulants, such as ephedra (ma huang), may reduce its effectiveness.

MUSCLE MAINTENANCE

Why is maintenance of muscle mass so important? Not only, as many people think, to make us look lean, fit, and strong (although those are all important). Instead, maintaining muscle mass also means that we maintain energy expenditure (muscle burns the vast majority of calories), reduce risk for osteoporosis (more muscle means denser bones), and protect ourselves from other chronic diseases such as heart disease, diabetes, and syndrome X.

So what supplements are effective for keeping us muscular? In answering this question, it is important to distinguish between the *maintenance* of muscle mass and the *enhancement* of muscle mass. On the one hand, there are a number of dietary supplements that can *maintain* muscle mass during various periods of high stress, but on the other hand, there are very few (perhaps none) that can *enhance* muscle mass (only high-dose anabolic steroids can do that effectively).

Numerous scientific and medical reports show quite clearly that high stress (such as extremes of exercise) and elevated cortisol levels lead to a dramatic loss of muscle tissue. High stress causes muscles to break down as a result of a number of factors, including elevated cortisol and suppressed levels of both testosterone and its precursor, DHEA (dehydroepiandrosterone). In cases of either high cortisol or low DHEA, or both, we know that reducing cortisol back down to normal levels and/or increasing DHEA back up to normal levels produces a dramatic effect on maintaining muscle mass. Importantly, however, it does not appear that reducing cortisol to below-normal levels or increasing DHEA to above-normal levels bears any beneficial effect on enhancing muscle mass (too bad for you bodybuilders out there).

The range of supplements that are commonly touted as *muscle maintainers* or *anticatabolics* (because they slow the catabolism, or breakdown, of muscle tissue) provide only a handful of substances that offer any good evidence of effectiveness: DHEA, zinc, cordyceps, CLA, and HMB. These are described below.

DHEA

DHEA (*dehydroepiandrosterone*) is a male sex hormone (androgenic hormone) produced in the adrenal glands, the same glands that produce cortisol. In the body, DHEA is converted into other hormones such as testosterone, estrogen, progesterone, or cortisol—so too much cortisol often means not enough DHEA. DHEA levels are known to decrease with age, particularly after the age of forty, but perhaps as early as ages twenty to thirty; therefore, dietary supplementation with DHEA is typically recommended to slow aging, improve memory, increase sex drive, alleviate depression, boost energy, promote weight loss, and build muscle mass.

DHEA supplementation, at 50–100 mg per day, has been shown to increase muscle mass and improve overall feelings of well-being among a group of forty- to seventy-year-old subjects who took the supplements for six months. Another small study (involving nine elderly men) showed a link between five months of DHEA supplementation (at 50 mg per day) and improvements in markers of immune-system function (lymphocytes, natural killer cells, and immunoglobulins). It is important for us to note, however, that the studies in which DHEA is effective in enhancing muscle mass and immune function have looked at subjects with low DHEA and testosterone levels to begin with; that means the DHEA supplements were restoring them to normal levels. Studies that have looked at healthy young men, with normal DHEA and testosterone levels, have shown no muscle-maintaining or immune-enhancing benefits, but instead an increase in estrogen levels—a bad thing because of the accompanying risk for increased cancer rates.

In people with low DHEA or low testosterone levels, both of which can result from chronic stress, DHEA supplements appear to be effective at doses ranging from 50 to 100 mg per day. DHEA supplements are one of the most popular muscle-building supplements among fitness enthusiasts. Most often sold in tablet or capsule form, DHEA is also sometimes added to protein powders and other products marketed for improving muscle mass. It is also a common ingredient in commercial products focused on anti-aging; its use in these is to counteract the well-known drop in DHEA levels that comes with age. Competitive athletes should be aware of the potential for DHEA supplementation to result in a positive drug test (for steroid use) at International Olympic Committee (IOC) and NCAA-sanctioned events.

Zinc

Zinc, which should already be a part of your comprehensive multimineral supplement, is an essential trace mineral that functions as part of about three hundred different enzymes. In terms of muscle maintenance, 60 percent of the body's zinc supply is stored in the muscles, and zinc is involved in numerous metabolic reactions related to testosterone production, wound healing, energy production, muscle growth, cellular repair, and reproductive function (especially male fertility). Even mild zinc deficiency has been associated with reduced testosterone levels, suppressed libido (sex drive), depressed immunity, decreased sperm count, and impaired memory. Perhaps the most popular claim for zinc is for its role in immunity; specifically, zinc delivered in lozenge form may interfere with the replication of the cold virus, which acts as a form of stress to the immune system (see also the discussion of selenium later in this chapter). Like vitamin C, zinc is an essential nutrient for optimal functioning of the immune system, and they both possess significant antiviral activity when consumed at elevated levels for a short period of time.

Luckily, dietary supplementation with zinc at levels of 15–45 mg per day has been shown to increase testosterone levels back to normal ranges, improve immune function, and restore sex drive. These levels of zinc should not pose any significant adverse side effects, but zinc supplementation needs to be balanced with copper intake (2 mg of copper for every 15 mg of zinc) to avoid the onset of copper deficiency caused by unbalanced zinc supplementation.

Cordyceps

Cordyceps (*Cordyceps sinensis*) is a Chinese mushroom that has been used for centuries to reduce fatigue, increase stamina, and improve lung function. Traditionally, it was harvested in the spring at elevations above fourteen thousand feet, restricting its availability to the privileged. You may remember news reports of cordyceps from a few years ago when a group of Chinese athletes began suddenly breaking world records in swimming and running events. Many of the athletes had been supplementing their diets with an extract from the cordyceps mushroom (along with turtle-blood soup and anabolic steroids).

Despite the steroid-laced Chinese athletes, several small-scale studies of a specific strain of cordyceps called *Cs-4* have shown improvements in lung function and suggested that athletes may benefit from an increased ability to take up and use oxygen. A handful of studies conducted in Chinese subjects have shown increases in libido (sex drive) and restoration of testosterone and DHEA levels (from low to normal) following cordyceps supplementation. Remember that during stressful events cortisol levels rise while DHEA levels drop. Using cordyceps as a way to normalize these suppressed

DHEA levels can help to modulate the cortisol:DHEA ratio within a lower (and healthier) range. Many of the claims for cordyceps parallel those of ginseng due to its reported effects on increasing energy levels, sex drive, and endurance performance.

Dietary supplements of cordyceps at levels of 2–4 grams per day are not associated with any significant side effects, although the possibility for a slight blood-thinning effect could reduce blood clotting somewhat. Cordyceps supplements are available primarily in powder and capsule forms at mainstream supplement stores, and the dried mushroom can occasionally be found in herbal pharmacies and from practitioners of traditional Chinese medicine (but it is very expensive in this form). Because more than two hundred different species of the cordyceps mushroom exist, it is important to look for the one on which the majority of the research has been conducted: the Cs-4 strain (typically standardized for mannitol content as a marker compound).

CLA

Conjugated linoleic acid (CLA) is found primarily in meat and dairy products, but the form of CLA used most commonly in dietary supplements is manufactured from vegetable oils such as sunflower oil. CLA is thought to increase the production of prostaglandins, which are derived from fatty-acid molecules and have been linked to an elevated synthesis of growth hormone and various anticatabolic effects (prevention of muscle breakdown) during periods of high stress. In athletes, increased growth-hormone levels are viewed as beneficial for promoting enhanced muscle growth and strength—but CLA does not appear to *enhance* muscle *growth* as effectively as it may be able to *suppress* muscle *loss* (at least in humans). CLA, via its involvement in prostaglandin metabolism, may also be able to increase blood circulation to the muscles and adipose tissue, an effect that has been suggested to improve muscle function and fat mobilization.

The majority of research on the dietary intake of CLA has been conducted in animals, but newer studies in humans are quite positive. Across the range of studies in rodents and in humans, CLA supplementation has been shown to reduce appetite, lower body weight, and enhance muscle maintenance, especially during active weight loss (viewed by the body as a powerful stressor).

Typical dosage recommendations are 3–6 grams per day. Most people ingest less than 1 gram per day from meat and dairy foods. Because CLA is an oil (liquid), supplements are provided almost exclusively in the form of softgel capsules; taking several large capsules per day is necessary to get an effective dose. However, a new, powdered form of CLA has recently been developed and should start showing up in powdered drink mixes and meal-replacement shakes in the near future.

HMB

HMB (*hydroxymethylbutyrate*) is a metabolite of the amino acid leucine, one of the branched-chain amino acids discussed earlier and which plays a role in regulating protein metabolism. In fact, HMB is thought to be the active form of leucine. HMB is found in the diet in small amounts in some protein-rich foods such as fish and milk. Depending on total protein and leucine intake, HMB production in the body may average about ¼–1 gram per day.

There is some evidence that HMB reduces muscle catabolism and may protect against muscle damage. NASA has evaluated HMB as a dietary approach to preventing the muscle wasting associated with prolonged space flight (talk about a stressful situation!). Exercise studies have shown that 1.5–3 grams of HMB daily during weight training can reduce muscle loss and muscle damage. No side effects have been reported in studies of HMB supplementation, but HMB can be quite expensive to take at these levels, making it less attractive to many people as a general muscle-maintenance supplement. Like DHEA, commercial sources of HMB are typically encapsulated powders marketed to bodybuilders and fitness enthusiasts, but HMB is also frequently added to protein powders and related muscle-building products.

IMMUNE ENHANCEMENT

The first thing to keep in mind about supporting the immune system with dietary supplements is that there is a huge difference
between chronic supplementation, which supports the immune
system on a regular basis, and acute supplementation, which bol-
sters immune-system activity to battle an existing infection. For
example, the popular immunostimulant herb echinacea appears to
be quite effective (when standardized for the right compounds) in
stimulating immune-system activity to battle a *new* infection, but
it is not recommended for prolonged or continuous use due to
concerns about cellular toxicity. Likewise, vitamin C and zinc
would be appropriate at low doses for chronic protection, whereas
higher levels are effective on a short-term basis for direct activity
against invading pathogens.

The primary key to bolstering immunity is, of course, to prevent infection in the first place. When it comes to prevention
(that is, to strengthening the immune system), it is always a good
idea to keep the immune system humming throughout the year,
not just when cold and flu season comes rumbling into town. To
that end, optimal support of immune-system function should
include managing stress, controlling cortisol levels, getting adequate amounts of exercise and rest, adhering to a balanced diet,
and reducing exposure to pathogens.

From a nutritional standpoint, a deficiency of any significant
nutrient can impair functioning of the immune system. Therefore,
just as it is a wise idea to take a daily multivitamin/multimineral
supplement to cover basic nutrient needs and to control cortisol
levels, it is also important to do so as part of immune-system support. Be sure to look for a multivitamin that supplies *at least* the
RDA levels for the essential nutrients. To round out your nutrient
armory, consider adding additional amounts of key amino acids
such as N-acetyl-cysteine (1–2 grams per day) or glutamine (1–5
grams per day), both of which have been linked to elevated
immune-system response. Finally, several immune-stimulating
herbs and herbal blends are available—the most effective of which

seem to be echinacea, goldenseal, and astragalus. These, and other immune-system boosters, are described below (except for astragalus, which is covered in Chapter 9).

Echinacea

With over three hundred scientific studies on its immune-enhancing effects, echinacea is "king" of the immune-function herbs. Across those studies, a number of reports show no benefits from echinacea supplementation, but among the two dozen or so largest and best-controlled studies, there is a significant reduction in reported cold symptoms and in the length of time required for subjects to become completely symptom free. It is important to note that the primary use of echinacea is for the acute, short-term treatment of the common cold—*not* for prolonged use (past a few weeks) as a general immune-system support. Also, individuals with autoimmune disorders, such as multiple sclerosis or rheumatoid arthritis, are generally advised to avoid using echinacea due to its immune-stimulating properties.

It is best to take echinacea immediately following acute exposure to an infected individual. For example, you should reach for the echinacea as soon as your sick Aunt Mary coughs on you.

When it comes to choosing an echinacea supplement, it is important to note that some alcohol extracts and some water extracts have been shown effective; however, there are also plenty of ineffective versions of both alcohol- and water-extracted echinacea supplements on the market. The one thing we know for sure is that the "pressed juice" (liquid) of the whole echinacea plant (flowers, leaves, stems, and roots), as well as a dried/encapsulated form of that pressed juice, is consistently effective in reducing cold symptoms and shortening the duration of infection. As soon as manufacturers try to extract or concentrate the alleged active ingredients in echinacea, the clinical effectiveness becomes much more difficult to define. That is, some extracts work and others do not, and nobody is sure why, but researchers in Kansas are close to figuring it out.

Goldenseal

Goldenseal is a popular herbal remedy for immune-system stimulation due to its high content of berberine. Because of the endangered status of goldenseal, however, many consumers (and supplement manufacturers) are turning to other berberine-containing herbs such as barberry and Oregon grape, which also appear to be quite effective alternatives for immune-system support. Berberine has been shown to block the adherence of various infectious bacteria (such as streptococci) to the body's respiratory linings; but berberine-containing herbs are known to cause uterine contractions, so they should be avoided during pregnancy.

Goldenseal supplements are found most commonly in combination with echinacea—with the best use of both herbs in acute situations (three weeks or less) to shorten the duration of a cold. Typical dosage recommendations for goldenseal root extract range from 250–500 mg (standardized to 5 percent total alkaloid levels).

Asian Mushrooms

A number of mushrooms are used in TCM to support immune-system strength. Among the more popular are shiitake, maitake, and reishi, all of which contain various polysaccharide (long chains of sugars) and amino-acid fractions (protein building blocks) that may help stimulate immune-cell activity and prepare the immune system for doing battle with invading pathogens. Although they are not completely understood, current theory suggests that the complex polysaccharides and small protein structures present in herbs such as astragalus and mushrooms such as reishi act as immunomodulators because of similarities between these compounds and the cellular surfaces of pathogenic bacteria, though the herbs lack the infectivity the pathogens have. This is a technical way of saying that these plant compounds are able to fool your immune system into mounting a more aggressive immune response than it ordinarily would against a simple cold virus or a cancer cell.

The optimal use of Asian mushrooms mirrors echinacea use: Add them to your supplement regimen at the earliest signs of infection. Asian mushrooms such as shiitake and maitake are now widely available in many grocery stores (and they taste great added to risotto or spaghetti sauce), but they are also showing up more and more as encapsulated powders for acute immune-system support. Reishi, on the other hand, is used more as a medicinal mushroom than as a food; traditional use focuses on suppression of tumor growth and cancer treatment. Although dried reishi mushrooms may be found in Chinese supermarkets, they are very tough (about the consistency of petrified wood) and require a lot of work to soften them for use in tea. Instead, reishi is probably best incorporated into a supplement regimen via a standardized extract that concentrates the polysaccharides into a more convenient (capsule) form. General dosage recommendations for Asian mushroom supplementation are in the range of 2–6 grams per day, with doses of the more concentrated reishi extracts in the range of 500–1,000 mg per day.

Probiotics and Prebiotics

Probiotics, also called *beneficial bacteria,* are quite effective for supporting immune function. The most popular varieties used in dietary supplements, *Lactobacillus acidophilus* and *Bifidobacteria bifidum,* have been shown in hundreds of studies to boost immune function via their effects on increasing white-blood-cell numbers, activity, and effectiveness. Used in conjunction with a few grams of *prebiotics* (indigestible carbohydrates that "feed" the growth of friendly bacteria in the intestines) such as fructo-oligosaccharides (FOS), probiotic organisms can displace certain pathogenic microbes in the intestines to prevent disease.

The strength of a probiotic supplement is measured in CFUs (colony-forming units) to designate the absolute number of viable bacteria in each capsule—but be sure to study the label, because many products report CFUs on a "per gram" basis even though each capsule may provide less than half that amount. When used as a treatment (such as to alleviate diarrhea), the recommended dose of probiotics is 10 billion CFUs per day, taken for three to seven days; daily dosage of probiotics when used as a preventive measure is lower, in the 2–4 billion range.

When choosing a probiotic supplement, it is very important to get one that actually provides viable organisms that can make it to your intestine and perform their functions in supporting gastro-intestinal health and immune-system support. The problem is that the majority of the probiotic products sitting on the shelf at your local pharmacy or supplement store are dead—and thus will pro-vide very few health benefits if you take them. Probiotics die as the result of heat, light, moisture, and age, each of which conspires to kill these beneficial bacteria before a user can get them into her or his body. The secret to choosing a probiotic supplement is to select one that is fresh (as far from the expiration date as possible), stored properly (away from light, heat, and moisture while on the shelf, and then kept in the refrigerator at home after being opened), and a blend of several strains of different bacteria (different strains can survive different extremes of temperature and other conditions).

Bioflavonoids

Bioflavonoids—such as quercetin, rutin, hesperidin, and a number of catechins and polyphenols found in green tea, grape seed, and pine-bark extracts—all possess powerful antioxidant functions that can both strengthen immune-system cells and protect healthy body tissues from damage. Taken separately, or in combination in mixed bioflavonoid complexes, these phytochemical compounds (substances naturally occurring in plants) can be taken at dosages of several hundred milligrams per day to help prevent infections and alleviate mild symptoms of colds, flu, and allergies.

Vitamin C

Vitamin C (discussed in more detail in Chapter 7) is the perennial immune booster and cold fighter. Despite the exaggerated old-wives' tales of vitamin C as a *prevention* against the common cold, it is clear that regular consumption of higher than RDA amounts of vitamin C (500 mg to 2 grams daily) can help reduce the *duration* and *severity* of colds. In fact, clinical studies now suggest that about 1 gram of vitamin C consumed on a regular basis throughout the cold and flu season can reduce cold incidence by about 20 percent and cold duration by almost 40 percent. Vitamin C can also act as a natural antihistamine to help open up congested airways. In some people, however, high doses (500 mg or more) can produce mild diarrhea or gas, so you may need to experiment to find the most effective dose for you. Do this by reducing your intake until symptoms disappear.

Vitamin A

Vitamin A is an effective immune-system nutrient because it helps keep bacteria and viruses from penetrating the protective mucous membranes of the mouth, nose, stomach, and lungs and thereby gaining a foothold in the body. Since vitamin A is a fat-soluble vitamin, people on low-fat diets may be limiting their consumption of foods rich in vitamin A (liver and dairy foods) and should consider a supplement. For men and postmenopausal women, vitamin A is considered relatively safe up to 25,000 IU (international units) per day. In pregnant women, or in those who could become pregnant, less than 10,000 IU per day is more prudent, as high doses of vitamin A are linked to birth defects and other damaging effects in the developing fetus. Any woman considering becoming pregnant should discuss vitamin A supplementation with her personal physician. A safer alternative may be to consider a mixed carotenoid supplement—because beta-carotene can be converted into vitamin A in the body—but only at levels required by the body.

Selenium

The trace mineral selenium is a building block of one of the body's key antioxidant enzymes, glutathione peroxidase (GPx). GPx is thought to also play a key role in helping immune-system cells protect the body from invading viruses and bacteria. Selenium has shown positive results as an important immune-system nutrient in studies of AIDS, chronic fatigue syndrome, and cancer (some forms of which may be caused by viruses). When selenium is combined with zinc, the two nutrients provide a boost to general immunity (see also the discussion of zinc earlier in this chapter).

Since few Americans get the recommended amounts of either selenium or zinc from their diets, a dietary supplement may be needed, especially during the cold and flu season. To achieve intake levels associated with enhanced immunity, consider a supplement providing selenium (200 mcg per day) and zinc (15–45 mg per day) together.

Summary

As you can see, the supplements summarized in this chapter are likely to be most effective when used to target specific instances of poor blood-sugar control, accelerated muscle loss, and suppressed immune-system function. As mentioned at the start of the chapter, you're more likely to get a bigger bang for your buck by controlling cortisol levels in the first place than by trying to reverse the detrimental effects of elevated cortisol on a piecemeal basis. It is interesting to note that the majority of the immune-system benefits delivered by dietary supplements are going to come from a multivitamin/multimineral supplement, which is also the foundation of a cortisol-control regimen, while the bulk of muscle maintenance effects and blood-sugar–control results will come from a specific cortisol-control regimen, as outlined in Chapter 8.

With all these separate recommendations, it is logical that you may feel a bit confused about how to put them into practice—but don't stress out about it! The next, and final, chapter pulls all of the preceding eleven chapters together into the simple plan, summarized in Chapter 5, called SENSE: stress management, exercise, nutrition, supplementation, and evaluation.

CHAPTER 12

Putting It All Together: The SENSE Program

You've heard it before—the familiar message that health experts (including your dear old grandmother) have been repeating for years: Get enough sleep, eat right, and exercise. Yes, it's a tired old mantra, but these three steps are probably the most effective tools available for combating stress and keeping cortisol levels from getting the best of us. Stress researchers from Yale to the University of California have shown over and over that the best way of managing stress, from both a physical and psychological perspective, is to adhere to the basic tenets of good health promotion—eat right, sleep, and exercise. (See how smart your grandma was?) Failure to do so, as we know by now, causes an elevation in cortisol levels and sets the stage for chronic diseases.

Unfortunately, when we are exposed to periods of heightened stress, what do we do? We do exactly the opposite of what we're supposed to. Instead of exercising, we stop our workout program, because stress makes us feel as if we simply don't have enough time. Instead of eating right, elevated cortisol levels make us hungry, so we grab something at the drive-through window. And instead of getting enough sleep to help our bodies counteract the debilitating effects of stress, we stay up late, wake up early, and suffer from restlessness and insomnia.

Researchers at the National Institutes of Health (NIH) have been studying the behavioral effects of heightened stress for more than thirty years. Their work shows quite clearly that stress causes us to undereat during the early stages of our stress response (maybe up to an hour), while our longer-term response to chronic stress, lasting from hours to days, is to overeat. This effect was confirmed in weight-loss centers around the country and the world after the September 11, 2001, terrorist attacks on the Pentagon and the World Trade Center. The resulting stress led many dieters to report stress-induced suppression of appetite, caused by feeling sick to their stomachs, followed some hours later by reports of stress-induced food binges, caused by a cortisol-stimulated appetite. NIH researchers have estimated that at least one-quarter of all Americans—more than sixty million people—will suffer an abnormal stress response to the events of September 11, which sets many of us up for increased risk of chronic diseases such as obesity, diabetes, heart disease, and others.

Enough doom and gloom. We know that stress is "bad" and we know that chronically elevated cortisol levels are "bad"—but what can we do about it? That's where the SENSE program comes in. SENSE, as you probably recall by now, stands for stress management, exercise, nutrition, supplementation, and evaluation.

STRESS MANAGEMENT

As mentioned in the early chapters, a variety of effective stress-management techniques exist that can be very helpful in controlling one's bodily responses to stressful situations. It is not, however, the focus of this book to highlight any specific stress-management techniques—for that, there are many excellent sources, a few of which are listed in the Resources section.

Instead, the entire category of stress management is broken down here into three simple categories: (1) Avoid stress, (2) manage stress, and (3) get enough sleep. To some readers, this may appear to be an overly simplistic approach to a topic as complex as stress management. Those readers are quite correct—but for the vast majority of people (your author included), these three simple steps will provide the biggest bang for the time they are prepared to devote to the specific practice of stress management (which is not a great deal of time).

Avoid Stress (Whenever You Can)

It probably comes as no surprise that the most effective stress-management technique is to simply avoid all those stressful situations in the first place. That way, you have no exposure to stress, no overactive stress response, and no increase in cortisol levels. Obviously, the goal of avoiding *all* stressful situations is unrealistic, but with proper planning, it may be possible to avoid *some* of them—or at least to plan effective strategies for dealing with the situations that cause you the most stress.

As an example, one of the things that causes me a great deal of stress is sitting in rush-hour traffic. My personal strategy to avoid this source of stress is to make sure I stay ahead of the traffic by leaving the house as early as possible in the morning and the office as early as possible in the evening. Of course, with two small children at home, it is often impossible to leave the house as early as planned, nor does the pile of work on my desk always allow me to leave the office as early as I wish. On those days, when my first-line stress-avoidance strategy of leaving early fails, I know I'll be sitting in traffic and I know I'll need to employ my backup plan, which is to listen to a book on tape. The book on tape allows me to avoid a personal source of stress because it enables me either to learn something new or to lose myself in a story—instead of stewing my way through a time-wasting traffic jam.

It is important to understand that each person will have a different strategy for avoiding their own personal stressors; the key is to find the plan (and a backup plan) that works best for you.

Manage Stress (As Effectively As You Can)

Obviously, if you can't avoid stress, then you've got to manage stress as effectively as possible. It might be instructive to review the discussion in Chapter 5 about the three mediating factors in the body's response to stress: whether there is any *outlet* for the stress, whether the stressor is *predictable,* and whether the individual thinks they have any *control* over the stressor.

Meditation, yoga, or getting in touch with your "inner self" may all be perfectly acceptable and beneficial outlets for stress, but managing stress is a very individualized concept, and a technique that reduces stress for one person may very well increase it for another. Readers who want to go beyond the approaches to stress management covered in this book are referred to the Resources chapter for a list of books that focus on a more emotional or psychological approach to stress management.

Get Some Sleep!

Yes, you say, it makes perfect sense that you need to spend enough time in bed when you're stressed; unfortunately, that stress also throws a great big monkey wrench into your normal sleep patterns. Not to mention the fact that our modern, Type C lifestyles have us living "24/7" schedules—so who's got time to sleep anyway? The main problem with this situation is that, aside from the well-known bad mood and inability to concentrate that we've all experienced from too few hours in the sack, sleep researchers have recently linked a chronic lack of sleep to increased appetite, problems with blood-sugar control, and a higher risk of diabetes and obesity—and chronically elevated cortisol is the obvious culprit. Researchers at both the University of Pennsylvania and the University of Chicago have shown that while too little sleep (six hours per night for a week) heightens an already revved-up stress response and keeps cortisol levels elevated, getting back into a more normal sleep pattern (eight hours per night) can reverse many of these detrimental changes and bring cortisol levels back to normal.

Getting more sleep, of course, is easier said than done, so the experts at the National Sleep Foundation recommend a few simple steps, like the ones listed below, for helping to get a person back on track to the eight hours most of us need each night:

- Establish a regular bedtime and a regular wake-up time— and stick to them for one week, even on the weekends (no matter how hard it is for the first few days). Sleep researchers tell us that within a week our body clocks will reset themselves to the new schedule.

- Do something calming in the hour or so before bedtime — such as relaxing with a book and a warm cup of chamomile tea, doing a crossword puzzle, or whatever else provides you with a few moments of peaceful reflection. My own getting-ready-for-bed ritual typically also includes a 100 mg dose of theanine (thirty to sixty minutes before I plan to climb under the covers), some light reading or a magazine to flip through, and a background of low-key jazz from the local public-radio station.

- Avoid exercise within three hours of bedtime. Exercise causes an increase in hormones, body temperature, and alertness—each of which will thwart efforts to fall asleep. For most people, exercising after work or even right after dinner (between 5:00 P.M. and 7:00 P.M.) is probably okay (assuming bedtime will be three to four hours later), because sufficient time is still allowed for the body to calm down and return to resting levels.

EXERCISE

Like getting enough sleep during stressful periods, getting enough exercise is another one of those no-brainers—but few of us follow through on what we know we should be doing. Ideally we've all experienced that feeling of postexercise relaxation that comes from elevated endorphins and lowered stress hormones. Aside from the feel-good, mind-clearing effects of exercise, however, are the obvious general health benefits for the heart and muscles, and also the general antistress benefits that help to control appetite, regulate blood sugar, curb overeating, and improve sleep.

The high-stress/low-sleep/no-exercise cycle is a vicious one— but breaking it, even by doing a small amount of exercise several days a week, can yield dramatic benefits. The key point here is that you don't need to become an Ironman triathlete or start training for a marathon. A simple game of racquetball, a walk around the block, or a quick circuit of sit-ups and push-ups before you head out the door to work will go a long way toward getting those cortisol levels back into a healthy range. Even light physical activity in small, manageable doses will trigger a cascade of stress-busting benefits, from lowering blood pressure to improving mood. See the Resources section for some excellent ideas to get you started on a regular stress-busting exercise program, and also review the list below to jump-start your thinking about ways to sneak small increments of exercise into your daily routine:

- At the mall or grocery store, add a few hundred yards of walking to your daily activity tally by parking in the middle or back of the lot instead of at the front.

- If you use public transportation, try riding your bike to the train station or bus stop, or park your car a few blocks away and walk the rest of the way to catch your ride.

- At the airport, be a rebel and take the stairs instead of the escalator (be sure to smile at the people on the escalator; you'll feel better just doing that).

- Put a basket on the front of your bicycle. You might look like Mary Poppins, but now you can use the bike to run short errands to the store.

- Instead of having a neighborhood kid (or your own kids) do your exercise for you, get out there yourself to mow the lawn, sweep the steps, rake the leaves, and shovel the driveway.

Jayne was about as Type C (high cortisol) as anyone you could imagine. An honor student and champion distance runner in college, she now worked for a large hospital group as a director of nursing. Among her fellow nurses Jayne was notorious for putting in long hours, taking paperwork home with her, and being on call at all hours of the day or night. Jayne considered herself to have a "high-energy" personality; she felt she thrived on the demands and stress that came with directing a large nursing group.

For six years Jayne did just fine. Despite the high-stress work that followed her home, and despite having chronically elevated cortisol levels from that high stress—as well as from inadequate sleep and poor diet—she seemed to be able to handle her stress load perfectly well. During that period, Jayne was promoted several times at work, maintained her athletic figure and healthy body weight from college, and enjoyed a loving relationship with her former college boyfriend, and now husband, *Jim*.

Everything in Jayne's life was going according to plan—everything was perfect—and then all hell broke loose. The straw that broke the camel's back, so to speak, was the birth of Jayne's first child. Having a baby was something that both Jayne and Jim had been planning and looking forward to since before they were married, so they were both well prepared mentally for the arrival of their new bundle of joy. The problem, however, was that Jayne was trying to maintain her pre-baby work schedule along with her new motherhood duties. Jim helped with the baby as much as possible, but his travel schedule as a district sales manager meant that he was out of town on business at least a few times each month, leaving Jayne to juggle work, day care, and nightly feedings for the baby. The combination of this being Jayne's first baby and her self-described tendency to be a "worrier" (about the baby, about her work, and about Jim when he was traveling), caused her to experience some of the highest stress levels—and highest cortisol levels—of her entire life. Couple those high stress levels with changes in her exercise program (rarely having the time) and in her diet (grabbing whatever junk food happened to be most convenient), and Jayne was on a crash course with cortisol.

Jayne's elevated cortisol levels manifested themselves primarily in the form of an inability to lose the "baby weight" she had gained during pregnancy, a growing struggle to stay focused on the complex tasks required of her at work, and great difficulty in falling asleep at night and then in getting back to sleep after waking with the baby.

Jayne started following the SENSE program with the primary goal of using it as a structure to control her diet and lose the excess pregnancy weight. As a former competitive athlete, she knew the importance of regular exercise for general health, but with the demands placed on her at home and work, there simply were not enough hours in the day to schedule what Jayne considered to be a worthwhile amount of exercise. Her idea of worthwhile exercise was to drive fifteen minutes to the gym, participate in a forty-five-minute high-intensity aerobic-dance class, stretch, shower, and then drive home. That's almost two hours out of her day; no wonder she had no time for exercise.

The first step, when it came to incorporating some exercise (the first E in SENSE) into her daily routine, was to get her to think about exercise in a different way. Over the next several weeks, Jayne began to sprinkle small amounts of exercise throughout the day—taking the stairs whenever possible at work, pushing her baby in his stroller when the weather was nice, and parking her car at the back of the parking lot and walking the hundred yards to the front door of the grocery store. Jayne even took her sprinkling of exercise to the extreme by performing a set of deep knee bends while her baby was swallowing between each spoonful of baby food. Suffice it to say that Jayne embraced the concept of sneaking exercise into her day—and even though she would have preferred to be out running five miles or sweating at the gym, she accepted the fact that this was as good as it was going to get at this point in her life.

In terms of nutrition, Jayne's greatest challenge was her constant snacking. Because she had difficulty planning the balanced meals she knew she should be eating, Jayne was in a constant state of "grab and go"—and there didn't appear to be any practical solution for alleviating that. Instead, the most practical solution for Jayne was to make each of those "grab and go" meals a more balanced blend of carbohydrates, proteins, fats, fiber, vitamins, and minerals. The most logical way to do that was to incorporate meal replacements, that is, shakes and energy bars. For Jayne, grabbing a shake for breakfast or a bar for the drive to work offered just the right amount of structure. Doing so enabled her to get the fuel she needed to keep her metabolism humming, it helped her control her blood sugar and banished her late-afternoon cravings for sweets, and it gave her the willpower she needed to resist sneaking to the fridge for a late-night snack after putting the baby to bed.

Perhaps the aspect of SENSE that made the most significant impact on Jayne's stress and cortisol levels was her incorporation of dietary supplements into her daily schedule. During her pregnancy she had already become accustomed to taking a daily multivitamin, so it was easy for her to continue this positive habit. In addition to her multi, Jayne also added a twice-daily theanine supplement (50 mg with breakfast and 100 mg before bed) and a midday dose of *Cordyceps sinensis* and American ginseng. The combination of cordyceps and ginseng provided the dual benefits of blood-sugar regulation (and added appetite control) along with an energy boost, without the side effects of stimulants. Theanine helped Jayne to stay calm and focused during the day (without drowsiness), while also helping her to sleep soundly during the night and fall *back* to sleep after getting up with the baby. The higher quality of sleep combined with heightened energy and mental focus during the day helped Jayne to regain her sense of relaxation and emotional balance.

In addition to these mental aspects of cortisol control, the exercise, nutrition, and supplements in Jayne's personalized SENSE plan helped her to modulate her blood-sugar levels, control her appetite, accelerate her fat metabolism, and lose the weight she had gained during pregnancy. In short, SENSE provided a simple and easy-to-follow framework for Jayne to use in getting her life back under control—and back to the place where she felt it should be.

NUTRITION

What is the first thing many of us do when the stress starts to pile up? We pile up our plates—and we usually do it with junk. Nothing stimulates our cravings for sugar, salt, and fat like a stressful event, but attempting to "eat your way out" is *not* the right approach. An entire book could be devoted to helping a person craft his or her own antistress diet (and many have been; see the Resources section for some recommended reading), but it's possible to get the most dramatic benefits from making a few small changes.

First, eat breakfast! Remember Mom telling you how breakfast was the most important meal of the day? Well, she was right—but not all breakfasts are created equal. Breakfast, like all your meals and snacks throughout the day, should be a blend of carbohydrates and protein, with a little bit of fat thrown in. Review Chapter 5 for a more detailed discussion of the ideal protein/fat/carbohydrate ratios, but a good rule of thumb is to compose each meal or snack by "fists." Here's how it works: Each meal (breakfast, lunch, and dinner) is made up of one fist-sized helping of carbohydrates (pasta, bread, cereal), one fist-sized helping of protein (meat, poultry, fish, tofu), and another fist or two of fruits and vegetables (an apple, a banana, a side salad). Each snack (one each between breakfast and lunch, between lunch and dinner, and between dinner and bedtime) should be built the same way, but the total size of a snack should be no larger than one fist.

Using this simple "fist" method does a few important things for your diet. Eating this way helps to control blood-sugar levels, regulate appetite, and maintain a high resting metabolic rate throughout the day. Eating this way also forces you to consume more fruits and vegetables, something the National Cancer Institute has been telling us to do for a long time (they recommend five daily servings of fruits and vegetables). Fruits and veggies are also rich in the vitamins and minerals our bodies need at higher levels during stressful times.

Want more specific guidance about what to eat? Flip to the Appendix (located after this chapter), which provides several daily food-selection plans for different calorie levels. A formula for estimating your caloric needs is also included.

If there was one thing in the world that caused *Marta* a high level of stress, it was her distress at her inability to lose those "last ten pounds" of body fat from around her hips and buttocks. Marta was a veteran of just about every fad diet in existence, but nothing seemed to work. As a self-described "stress monster," Marta was attracted to the SENSE program because it combined both physical and mental aspects of health. Marta felt that she needed help to balance her eating habits with her exercise regimen (don't we all), but she was intimidated by the "no pain, no gain" mentality that she encountered at her local gym. As someone who was also prone to anxiety attacks, the last thing the Type C Marta needed was a Type A fitness trainer pushing her through an aggressive exercise regimen. Instead, Marta opted for an approach to exercise that helped her to feel more relaxed, less stressed, and more focused.

That approach to exercise was to largely "forget about it" and focus on simply getting in as many miles of walking as possible in a given week. Marta bought a small pedometer to record the number of steps she took each day—and she made it her goal to record as many steps as possible. Taking the "forget about it" approach to exercising, Marta removed a primary source of stress (and excess cortisol) from her life. Marta's newfound cortisol control allowed her body to readjust its metabolic profile, with tighter blood-sugar control, controlled appetite, and accelerated fat metabolism the primary outcomes that inched Marta toward her ultimate goal of saying good-bye to those "last ten pounds" for good.

In place of focusing on the exercise portion of the SENSE program, Marta chose to focus her efforts on the nutrition (N), supplement (S), and evaluation (E) aspects of the plan. In terms of nutrition, Marta went on an aggressive regimen of meal replacements (plus a daily multivitamin/multimineral supplement). Shakes and bars replaced breakfast, lunch, and two snacks for four weeks; a healthy dinner was the only "real" meal that Marta prepared for the entire month. Following that initial four-week period, Marta reevaluated her efforts and her goals. She had lost a little more than five pounds of body weight—and a body-fat analysis indicated that 80 percent of her weight loss was from fat—so Marta was about halfway to her goal and certainly on the right track.

The only complaint she noted during her first four weeks was a craving for sweets in the late afternoon and in the evening before bed, so she felt that perhaps she needed to increase her total calorie consumption by just a bit in the next phase (six weeks). This slight increase in calorie consumption came from incorporating more "real" foods into her diet. Dinner remained the same balanced meal of one fist-sized piece of protein (such as salmon), one fist-sized serving of carbohydrates (such as rice), and two fist-sized servings of salad or steamed vegetables. But Marta now followed the same balancing guidelines (while cutting the fist-sized portions in half) when she made her lunchtime sandwich (whole-grain roll, turkey, lettuce, tomato, sprouts, and low-fat mayo). She also added a twice-daily supplement of 100 mcg of chromium, 10 mcg of vanadium, and 15 mg of banaba leaf extract (at lunch and dinner only) to help control her blood sugar and her cravings for sweets in late afternoon and evening.

During this six-week period, Marta noted that her cravings for sweets had vanished. But even more important was her continued weight loss, which topped out at twelve pounds lost (90 percent of it from body fat) in just ten weeks. Marta had exceeded her weight-loss goals—an objective she had failed to achieve on numerous occasions in the past—and the primary difference between then and now was the more relaxed and balanced approach she'd followed.

Now came another evaluation period. This time Marta needed to decide whether to try to continue with additional weight loss or simply attempt to maintain what she had already accomplished. Knowing that weight *maintenance* can be much more difficult for many people than the initial weight *loss*, Marta was feeling a bit apprehensive about the possibility that she might gain back all of her lost weight. As a way to counteract her growing anxiety (which could increase her cortisol levels and set the stage for weight regain), she continued with a daily nutrition program that looked like this:

Breakfast: Meal-replacement shake plus multivitamin/mineral supplement (250 calories)

Morning snack: Energy bar (160 calories)

Lunch: Turkey sandwich plus chromium/vanadium/banaba supplement (380 calories)

Afternoon snack: Handful of nuts and glass of water (180 calories)

Dinner: Grilled chicken with steamed rice and vegetables plus chromium/vanadium/banaba supplement (520 calories)

Evening snack: Chocolate milk with piece of fruit (240 calories)

Total calories: 1,730

In addition to her balanced nutrition regimen, Marta added a twice-daily supplement of magnolia bark extract to her morning and evening snacks. The mild antianxiety effects of magnolia helped Marta to stay focused and remain calm about her switch to a slightly higher-calorie weight-maintenance regimen—so she didn't get stressed out and her cortisol levels stayed in their normal ranges.

To many of her friends, Marta is now one of those "lucky" people who is able to "effortlessly" maintain her new, slimmer figure without much attention to diet or exercise. More than once she has been told that she must have "good genes" to be able to eat the way she does (to some, it looks as if she eats all the time), take a laissez-faire attitude toward high-intensity exercise, and generally seem unconcerned and relaxed about the whole public furor over body weight.

SUPPLEMENTATION—LEVEL I

Although this book focuses a great deal on controlling the stress response and cortisol levels using dietary supplements, it is important to emphasize that supplements fall *fourth* in the whole scheme of things—behind stress management, regular exercise, and optimal nutrition. From a practical point of view, however, many of us simply do not have the ability, time, or inclination to live the "perfect" antistress lifestyle—and in those situations, supplements play a more prominent role.

So, *after* doing what you can do in terms of stress avoidance/management, getting adequate amounts of sleep and exercise, and eating a balanced diet, *then* turn your attention to using dietary supplements to help control cortisol. When you begin to focus on the supplement side of things, it makes sense to approach them step by step, as follows:

Step 1

Avoid excessive doses of supplements that can increase cortisol levels (Chapter 6). These tend to be ingredients that fall into the category of herbal stimulants, and are often found in weight-loss and appetite-suppressant products. These supplements, *when used at appropriate doses*, certainly appear to offer a small benefit for promoting weight loss by controlling appetite, increasing energy levels, and boosting thermogenesis (calorie burning). When used in excessive doses, however, they will increase cortisol levels, disrupt blood-sugar levels, increase appetite, and sabotage efforts at long-term weight control.

Step 2

Take a comprehensive multivitamin/multimineral supplement (Chapter 7). In particular, the supplement you choose should provide adequate amounts of the most important antistress nutrients that are needed at increased levels during periods of high stress: vitamin C, magnesium, calcium, and the B-complex vitamins. Your multivitamin/multimineral supplement will provide the foundation of your cortisol-control supplement regimen, so the more comprehensive it is, providing the full range of essential nutrients, the better.

Step 3

Focus on targeted cortisol-modulating supplements (Chapter 8). This is where you'll be able to make the most dramatic gains toward maintaining healthy cortisol levels using supplements. Of the many supplements that may play a role in modulating the stress response and controlling cortisol levels, the most direct and promising benefits are likely to come from beta-sitosterol (BS), magnolia bark, epimedium, and theanine.

This is as far as most people will need to go in terms of using supplements to help control cortisol levels. When these are used in the context of the entire SENSE program, they help keep cortisol levels in a healthy range so that you reap the long-term health benefits.

SUPPLEMENTATION—LEVEL II

Each of the next three steps in the supplementation regimen should be viewed as a temporary "control point" designed to rebalance the stress response. The supplements addressed in this section (described in detail in Chapters 9–11) are intended to be used only in specific cases of heightened stress (adaptogens, Chapter 9), for targeted antianxiety/antidepression effects (relaxation and calming supplements, Chapter 10), and when stress has gained the upper hand and you are suffering from insomnia, muscle loss, or immune-system suppression (metabolic-support supplements, Chapter 11).

Step 4

Consider adding "reinforcement" supplements against stress in the form of adaptogens (Chapter 9). Most people will get all the cortisol control they need through stress management, exercise, nutrition, and the first three steps of the supplement regimen. However, during specific periods of particularly high stress, a temporary adaptogen regimen (for example, ginseng and related supplements used for a couple weeks to a few months) may help control cortisol and thus fight fatigue and related stress symptoms in some people.

Step 5

Use relaxation and calming supplements to fight depression, insomnia, and stress (Chapter 10). In some cases, stress can get the best of us and require us to go beyond cortisol control. In these situations, you'll still be using each of the preceding steps in the SENSE program, but periods of especially high stress can lead to bouts of depression, anxiety, and insomnia. In these situations, the targeted cortisol-control supplements (outlined in Step 3 above) may be enough for some people, while others can benefit from a more specific herbal antidepressant (St. John's wort, SAM-e, or 5-HTP), antianxiety supplement (kava kava or gotu kola), or sleep aid (valerian or melatonin). As you become better able to control your stress response and modulate your cortisol levels, your need for these calming supplements is likely to be reduced.

Step 6

As outlined in Chapter 11, use other temporary support supplements for blood-sugar control (chromium, vanadium, banaba, and gymnema), muscle maintenance (DHEA, HMB, CLA, zinc, and cordyceps), and immune-system support (echinacea, vitamin C, selenium, probiotics, and others). As each of these conditions resolves itself, benefits can be maintained by using Steps 1 to 3 in the supplementation regimen.

> After learning about the detrimental health effects of chronically elevated cortisol, *Mario* joked that cortisol was his middle name—but he was serious about his desire to get his cortisol

levels under control. As a long-haul truck driver, Mario experienced the quadruple threat of high stress (time pressure to deliver his loads on time), inadequate exercise, poor nutrition, and irregular sleep patterns. As a textbook case for elevated cortisol levels, Mario was certainly about as extreme as they come.

On the stress-management end of things, Mario had a heck of a long way to go. As an extreme Type C personality, his highest cortisol exposure generally occurred during traffic jams, when he sat and virtually boiled in his own stress hormones. Mario's chief problem with traffic was that it kept him from meeting his tight schedule—and consequently he felt helpless and stressed whenever the traffic slowed to a crawl. After he tried a number of stress-management approaches (breathing exercises, positive imagery, music, books on tape, and others), the solution that finally worked for Mario was to talk to his family and friends on his cellular phone. As it turns out, part of the reason traffic caused Mario to experience such high stress was because he felt that it was another obstacle keeping him from spending time with his loved ones (and an obstacle that he could do little to influence). As a result, when the traffic slowed, Mario's stress increased—and so did his cortisol, his cholesterol, his appetite, and his waistline. The cell phone, along with unlimited long-distance minutes and a hands-free attachment to allow him to keep both hands on the wheel, allowed Mario to stay in touch with his wife, kids, and friends—and became a significant destress mechanism whenever he felt that he might be delayed. Even a conversation lasting a few minutes was enough for Mario and his family to stay mentally and emotionally connected during his frequent extended trips.

Now that the primary source of Mario's stress was identified and partially controlled, our attention turned to giving him a "supercharge" in terms of targeted cortisol control. Because his need to stay alert during the day was literally a matter of life and death (you don't want a drowsy driver behind the wheel of an eighteen-wheeler traveling at seventy miles per hour), some of the traditional antistress supplements (kava, valerian, melatonin) were ruled out because of their sedating effects. Instead, Mario started using theanine in the evening (200 mg taken as soon as he pulled his truck over for the night) as a way to relax him and help him fall asleep faster and stay asleep through the night. A significant side benefit of theanine was that he felt no "morning after" effects such as sluggishness or sleepiness, so he woke up refreshed and ready to face the long day ahead. Besides Mario's reports that he was feeling better (with more energy and clearer thinking), the increase in the quantity and quality of his sleep helped his body to better regulate its own cortisol levels (they slowly fell during the evening hours).

The second phase of supplementation for Mario was his incorporation of a daily multivitamin/multimineral along with a phosphatidylserine (PS) supplement in the morning and a beta-sitosterol (BS) supplement (also known as *phytosterols*) in the evening. The multi provided a general antistress foundation on which the PS and BS could begin to control cortisol levels. The morning dosing of PS took advantage of its dual effects in controlling cortisol and boosting brainpower and concentration (nice side effects for a truck driver in an unfamiliar city). The evening dosing of BS produced the dual effects of controlling cortisol and reducing cholesterol levels (Mario's largest and fattiest meal of the day was almost always dinner eaten at a roadside diner). The cholesterol-lowering effect of BS occurs at a much higher level (about 3 grams per day) than the cortisol-controlling effects (60–120 mg per day), but BS is perfectly safe, and four large capsules at dinner were not much of an inconvenience to Mario—especially given the fact that BS can block a large amount of cholesterol from being absorbed.

Mario enjoyed success in controlling his primary sources of cortisol overexposure (stressing out about traffic delays and getting inadequate sleep), but what about his diet and exercise patterns? It might surprise you that Mario's strategy in these areas was to do very little at all. We learned early on that a strict diet and exercise regimen was not only unrealistic for Mario's work and travel schedule, but it would also have represented an additional source of daily stress for him to deal with. Instead, the exercise piece of the puzzle was limited to walking on as many days of the week as possible when he was at home with his family (walks around the neighborhood became a sort of family event). The nutrition part of SENSE was also quite limited in its scope; it centered on counteracting Mario's tendency to snack on convenience foods from the cab of his truck. To this end, Mario agreed to focus his snacking on balanced foods—so donuts were replaced by whole-grain bagels with peanut butter, cupcakes were replaced by energy bars containing both carbohydrates and protein, and potato chips were replaced by a handful of mixed nuts.

After just a few days on the SENSE program, Mario noticed an immediate change in how he felt; the key benefits were sounder sleep, more energy, and a clearer mind. Within two weeks, Mario's appetite and eating habits came back into balance and he was able to start focusing on getting his body weight under control. Even without a "perfect" diet and exercise regimen, the fact that Mario had regained control over his body's stress response and cortisol levels made it possible for him to lose five inches off his waistline in a little less than six months. Mario still has a long way to go to get down to his ideal body weight, but with his cortisol-control issues out of the way he is headed in the right direction.

EVALUATION

It is important to keep in mind that neither one's stress levels nor the body's response to stress is a constant. Instead, there will be periods in each of our lives when we experience more stress or less stress—just as there will be times when we feel as if we can withstand stress better than other times. Accordingly, the last step in the SENSE program, evaluation, reminds us that we need to alter our exercise patterns, nutrient intake, and supplementation regimen according to our exposure to stress. For example, regular exercise and a balanced diet are always going to be important, but they become even more so during stressful times. Skipping breakfast during a period of low stress isn't ideal, but it isn't going to kill you. Skip that balanced breakfast during a high-stress period, however, and you're setting yourself up for poor blood-sugar control, surges in appetite, and feelings of fatigue—each of which will be even more pronounced because of your high-stress profile.

So how do you evaluate your current stress profile? Take the Stress Self-Test included in the Preface to get a good baseline gauge of your stress exposure and your cortisol levels—and then take it again every three months to reevaluate where you stand. Are you experiencing higher than normal stress levels? If so, then your cortisol levels are likely to be elevated, and you need to be especially careful about following each step of the SENSE program to keep them within a healthy range. Or are you enjoying an inter-lude that's relatively stress-free and tranquil? Then perhaps you can be less vigilant about using the Level II supplements, and relax and take pleasure in the welcome fruits of the healthy life-style you've created by following the sound stress-management, sleep, exercise, nutritional, and supplementation habits promoted by the SENSE plan. And once you've reached this point, having created these healthy new habits and having witnessed how they've benefited you, you'll be more motivated than ever to maintain them as part of your daily life.

Summary

I hope this book has made clear that cortisol is a necessary hormone, but also that cortisol levels elevated too high for too long will leave you feeling bad and looking bad, and put you on the fast track toward a long list of chronic diseases. Those conditions run the gamut from simple feelings of fatigue and forgetfulness to more serious debilitations such as obesity, diabetes, cancer, cardiovascular disease, and Alzheimer's disease.

The good news, however, is that following the SENSE program outlined in this book can help control your body's response to your many daily stressors, so that cortisol levels are maintained in a healthier range. Using the SENSE program will help you lose weight, maintain muscle mass, boost energy levels, reduce illness, increase brainpower, and enhance your sex drive.

As the scientific and medical research continues to advance linking cortisol and disease, additional wisdom will undoubtedly be discovered that we can all incorporate into our personal SENSE programs. I wish you the best in doing so, and in maintaining healthy cortisol levels and optimizing your long-term health.

Daily Food Plans

A rough rule of thumb for calculating daily caloric needs is to assume you need 10 calories for every pound of body weight. Therefore, a 120-pound woman might follow the 1,200-calorie plan included below, and a 200-pound man might choose the 2,000-calorie plan. Exercise will require that more calories be added; a rule of thumb here is to add 100 calories for every mile walked or jogged.

Instructions: Find the appropriate table (calorie level and meal). For your meal, choose one item from each row (A, B, C, etc.). Choose no more than one item from the column labeled "calorie dense," and no more than one from the column labeled "calorie moderate."

A sample breakfast at the 1,200-calorie level might look like this:

- ½ plain bagel (row A, calorie light)

- 1 oz. granola cereal (row B, calorie dense)

- 1 banana (row C, calorie moderate)

Daily Food-Selection Plan: 1,200 Calories

Breakfast

Choose one item from row A, one from row B, and one from row C. Choose no more than one item from the column labeled "calorie dense," and no more than one item from the column labeled "calorie moderate."

	Calorie Light	Calorie Moderate	Calorie Dense
A	• 1 slice French toast with syrup • 2 small pancakes with syrup • 1 waffle with syrup • ½ plain bagel, any type • 1 plain English muffin • 2 slices plain toast	• ½ slice French toast with syrup and butter or margarine • 1 small pancake with syrup and butter or margarine • ½ waffle with syrup and butter or margarine • ¼ bagel, any type, with cream cheese • ½ English muffin with butter, margarine, or peanut butter • 1 slice toast with butter and jelly • ½ sweet roll	• 1 biscuit with butter or margarine • ½ croissant with butter or margarine or 1 plain croissant • ½ danish • ½ donut, any type
B	• 1 package cream of wheat, instant oatmeal, or other hot cereal	• 2 oz. cold cereal (bran, corn, or wheat flakes, wheat squares, etc.) with 6 oz. skim milk and fruit	• 1 oz. granola-type or sugar-coated cereal with 6 oz. skim milk
C	• 1 piece of fresh fruit (apple, orange, kiwi, grapefruit) • 5 oz. canned fruit in juice or light syrup	• 1 banana • 3 oz. canned fruit in heavy syrup	• 1 oz. coconut, dates, dried fruit, prunes, or raisins

Lunch

Choose one item from row A, one from row B, one from row C, and an afternoon snack from row D. Choose no more than one item from the column labeled "calorie dense," and no more than one item from the column labeled "calorie moderate."

	Calorie Light	Calorie Moderate	Calorie Dense
A	Sandwich with as many vegetables as you want and: • 91% fat-free meat (2 slices) • grilled fish • tuna (in water) • turkey breast • vegetarian	Sandwich with as many vegetables as you want and: • 82–90% fat-free lunch meat (1 slice)	• Croissant sandwich with 1 slice of 91% fat-free meat • ½ meatball sub • ½ BLT with light mayo • ½ of any sandwich with full-fat mayo or cheese • 1 single-patty hamburger
B	• Large garden salad (6 oz.) with no dressing or with fat-free dressing	• Medium garden salad (3 oz.) with light salad dressing and croutons or olives	• Small garden salad with regular, Caesar, or oil dressing
C	8 oz.: • Apple juice or cider • Grapefruit juice • Orange juice • V-8 or tomato juice	5 oz.: • Cranberry juice (or other cran-juice) • Pineapple juice • Prune juice	• 2 oz. coconut milk
D	• 6 oz. nonfat cottage (or other) cheese or low-fat yogurt • ½ Powerbar or Breakbar	• 4 oz. low-fat frozen yogurt • ¼–½ energy bar*	• 2 oz. any full-fat cheese

* Choose an energy bar that provides a blend of protein, carbohydrates, fat, and fiber (such as Clif Bar, Balance Bar, etc.).

Dinner

Choose one item from row A, one from row B, one from row C, one from row D, and a nighttime snack from row E. Choose no more than one item from the column labeled "calorie dense," and no more than one item from the column labeled "calorie moderate."

	Calorie Light	Calorie Moderate	Calorie Dense
A	• Large garden salad (6 oz.) with no dressing or with fat-free dressing	• Medium garden salad (3 oz.) with light dressing and croutons or olives	• Small garden salad with regular, Caesar, or oil dressing
B	3 oz. any 90% fat-free (or better) meat, including: • Crab, lobster, shrimp (not fried) • Most types of broiled fish or other seafood • Poultry (white meat, no skin)	2 oz. any 82% fat-free meat, including: • Beef flank steak • Lean lamb • Pork tenderloin • Poultry (dark meat, no skin) • Regular ham • Veal	1 oz. any meat less than 82% fat-free, including: • Pork chops • Beef ribs • Fried chicken • Fried fish • Hotdog, sausage, or kielbasa • Poultry with skin
C	• 1 slice whole-grain bread • 1 whole-grain roll	• ½ slice whole-grain bread with butter or margarine • ½ croissant	• ¼ oz. nuts, seeds, or crackers
D	• Your fill of any vegetable (no butter, margarine, or cheese sauce)	• Your fill of any vegetable (no butter, margarine, or cheese sauce)	• 2 oz. vegetables, deep fried or with butter, margarine, or cheese sauce
E	• 1 piece of fresh fruit • 6 oz. jello • 2 Popsicles • 1 low-cal ice cream bar • ½ cup low-cal pudding	• 4–6 oz. low-fat frozen yogurt • 1 frozen fudge pop • ¼ cup regular pudding • ½ cup sherbet	• 1 oz. (small slice) of cake, pie, or pastry • 1 oz. chocolate • 1 small scoop of reduced-fat ice cream • 2 small chocolate-chip cookies • 3 Fig Newtons

Daily Food-Selection Plan: 1,400 Calories

Breakfast

Choose one item from row A, one item from row B, and two items from row C (one with breakfast and one as a mid-morning snack). Choose no more than one item from the column labeled "calorie dense," and no more than one item from the column labeled "calorie moderate."

	Calorie Light	Calorie Moderate	Calorie Dense
A	• 1 slice French toast with syrup • 2 small pancakes with syrup • 1 waffle with syrup • ½ plain bagel, any type • 1 plain English muffin • 2 slices plain toast	• ½ slice French toast with syrup and butter or margarine • 1 small pancake with syrup and butter or margarine • ½ waffle with syrup and butter or margarine • ¼ bagel, any type, with cream cheese • ½ English muffin with butter, margarine, or peanut butter • 1 slice toast with butter and jelly • ½ sweet roll	• 1 biscuit with butter or margarine • ½ croissant with butter or margarine or 1 plain croissant • ½ danish • ½ donut, any type
B	• 1 package cream of wheat, instant oatmeal, or other hot cereal	• 2 oz. cold cereal (bran, corn, or wheat flakes, wheat squares, etc.) with 6 oz. skim milk and fruit	• 1 oz. granola-type or sugar-coated cereal with 6 oz. skim milk
C	• 1 piece of fresh fruit (apple, orange, kiwi, grapefruit) • 5 oz. canned fruit in juice or light syrup	• 1 banana • 3 oz. canned fruit in heavy syrup	• 1 oz. coconut, dates, dried fruit, prunes, or raisins

Lunch

Choose one item from row A, one from row B, one from row C, and an afternoon snack from row D. Choose no more than one item from the column labeled "calorie dense," and no more than one item from the column labeled "calorie moderate."

	Calorie Light	Calorie Moderate	Calorie Dense
A	Sandwich with as many vegetables as you want and: • 91% fat-free meat (2–3 slices) • grilled fish • tuna (in water) • turkey breast • vegetarian	Sandwich with as many vegetables as you want and: • 82–92% fat-free lunch meat (1–2 slices)	• Croissant sandwich with 1 slice of 91% fat-free meat • ½ meatball sub • ½ BLT with light mayo • ½ of any sandwich with full-fat mayo or cheese • 1 single-patty hamburger
B	• Large garden salad (6 oz.) with no dressing or with fat-free dressing	• Medium garden salad (3 oz.) with light salad dressing and croutons or olives	• Small garden salad with regular, Caesar, or oil dressing
C	8 oz.: • apple juice or cider • grapefruit juice • orange juice • V-8 or tomato juice	5 oz.: • cranberry juice (or other cran-juice) • pineapple juice • prune juice	• 2 oz. coconut milk
D	• 6–8 oz. nonfat cottage (or other) cheese or low-fat yogurt • 1 Powerbar or Breakbar	• 4–6 oz. low-fat frozen yogurt • ½ energy bar*	• 2 oz. any full-fat cheese

* Choose an energy bar that provides a blend of protein, carbohydrates, fat, and fiber (such as Clif Bar, Balance Bar, etc.).

Dinner

Choose one item from row A, one from row B, one from row C, one from row D, and a nighttime snack from row E. Choose no more than one item from the column labeled "calorie dense," and no more than one item from the column labeled "calorie moderate."

	Calorie Light	Calorie Moderate	Calorie Dense
A	• Large garden salad (6 oz.) with no dressing or fat-free dressing	• Medium garden salad (3 oz.) with light salad dressing and croutons or olives	• Small garden salad with regular, Caesar, or oil dressing
B	4 oz. any 90% fat-free (or better) meat, including: • crab, lobster, shrimp (not fried) • most types of broiled fish or other seafood • poultry (white meat, no skin)	3 oz. any 82% fat-free meat, including: • beef flank steak • lean lamb • pork tenderloin • poultry (dark meat, no skin) • regular ham • veal	2 oz. any meat less than 82% fat-free, including: • pork chops • beef ribs • fried chicken • fried fish • hotdog, sausage, or kielbasa • poultry with skin
C	• 2 slices whole-grain bread • 2 whole-grain rolls	• 1 slice whole-grain bread with butter or margarine • ½ croissant	
D	• Your fill of any vegetable (no butter, margarine, or cheese sauce)	• Your fill of any vegetable (no butter, margarine, or cheese sauce)	• 2 oz. vegetables deep fried or with butter, margarine, or cheese sauce
E	• 1 piece of fresh fruit • 6 oz. jello • 2 Popsicles • 1 low-cal ice cream bar • ½ cup low-cal pudding	• 4–6 oz. low-fat frozen yogurt • 1 frozen fudge pop • ¼ cup regular pudding • ½ cup sherbet	• 1 oz. (*small* slice) of cake, pie, or pastry • 1 oz. chocolate • 1 small scoop of reduced-fat ice cream • 2 small chocolate-chip cookies • 3 Fig Newtons

Daily Food-Selection Plan: 1,600 Calories

Breakfast

Choose one item from row A, one from row B, and two from row C (one with breakfast and one as a mid-morning snack). Choose no more than one item from the column labeled "caloric dense," and no more than one item from the column labeled "calorie moderate."

	Calorie Light	Calorie Moderate	Calorie Dense
A	• 2 slices French toast with syrup • 3 pancakes with syrup • 2 waffles with syrup • 1 whole plain bagel, any type • 2 plain English muffins • 4 slices plain toast	• 1 slice French toast with syrup and butter or margarine • 2 pancakes with syrup and butter or margarine • 1 waffle with syrup and butter or margarine • ½ bagel, any type, with cream cheese • 1 English muffin with butter, margarine, or peanut butter • 2 slices toast with butter and jelly • 1 sweet roll	• 2 biscuits with butter or margarine • 1 croissant with or without butter or margarine • 1 danish • 1 donut, any type
B	• 1 package cream of wheat, instant oatmeal, or other hot cereal	• 2 oz. cold cereal (bran, corn, or wheat flakes, wheat squares, etc.) with 6 oz. skim milk and fruit	• 1 oz. granola-type or sugar-coated cereal with 6 oz. skim milk
C	• 1 piece fresh fruit (apple, orange, kiwi, grapefruit) • 5 oz. canned fruit in juice or light syrup	• 1 banana • 3 oz. canned fruit in heavy syrup	• 1 oz. coconut, dates, dried fruit, prunes, or raisins

Lunch

Choose one item from row A, one from row B, one from row C, and an afternoon snack from row D. Choose no more than one item from the column labeled "calorie dense," and no more than one item from the column labeled "calorie moderate."

	Calorie Light	Calorie Moderate	Calorie Dense
A	Sandwich with as many vegetables as you want and: • 91% fat-free meat (4 slices) • grilled fish • tuna (in water) • turkey breast • vegetarian	Sandwich with as many vegetables as you want and: • 82–92% fat-free regular lunch meat (2 slices)	• Croissant sandwich with 1 slice low-fat meat • ½ meatball sub • ½ BLT with light mayo • ½ any sandwich with full-fat mayo or cheese • 1 single-patty hamburger
B	• Large garden salad (6 oz.) with no dressing or with fat-free dressing	• Medium garden salad (3 oz.) with light salad dressing and croutons or olives	• Small garden salad with regular, Caesar, or oil dressing
C	8 oz.: • apple juice or cider • grapefruit juice • orange juice • V-8 or tomato juice	5 oz.: • cranberry juice (or other cran-juice) • pineapple juice • prune juice	• 2 oz. coconut milk
D	• 8 oz. nonfat cottage (or other) cheese or low-fat yogurt • 1 Powerbar or Breakbar	• 6 oz. low-fat frozen yogurt • ½ energy bar*	• 2–4 oz. any full-fat cheese

* Choose an energy bar that provides a blend of protein, carbohydrates, fat, and fiber (such as Clif Bar, Balance Bar, etc.).

Dinner

Choose one item from row A, one from row B, one from row C, one from row D, and a nighttime snack from row E. Choose no more than one item from the column labeled "calorie dense," and no more than one item from the column labeled "calorie moderate."

	Calorie Light	Calorie Moderate	Calorie Dense
A	• Large garden salad (6 oz.) with no dressing or with fat-free dressing	• Medium garden salad (3 oz.) with light salad dressing and croutons or olives	• Small garden salad with regular, Caesar, or oil dressing
B	6 oz. any 90% fat-free (or better) meat, including: • crab, lobster, shrimp (not fried) • most types broiled fish or other seafood • poultry (white meat, no skin)	4 oz. any 82% fat-free meat, including: • beef flank steak • lean lamb • pork tenderloin • poultry (dark meat, no skin) • regular ham • veal	2.5 oz. any meat less than 82% fat-free, including: • pork chops • beef ribs • fried chicken • fried fish • hotdog, sausage, or kielbasa • poultry with skin
C	• 2 slices whole-grain bread • 2 whole-grain rolls	• 1 slice whole-grain bread with butter or margarine • 1 croissant	• ½ oz. nuts, seeds, or crackers
D	• Your fill of any vegetable (no butter, margarine, or cheese sauce)	• Your fill of any vegetable (no butter, margarine, or cheese sauce)	• 3 oz. vegetables deep fried or with butter, margarine, or cheese sauce
E	• 1 piece fresh fruit • 6 oz. jello • 2 Popsicles • 1 low-cal ice cream bar • ½ cup low-cal pudding	• 4–6 oz. low-fat frozen yogurt • 1 frozen fudge pop • ¼ cup regular pudding • ½ cup sherbet	• 1 oz. (*small* slice) of cake, pie, or pastry • 1 oz. chocolate • 1 small scoop reduced-fat ice cream • 2 small chocolate-chip cookies • 3 Fig Newtons

Daily Food-Selection Plan: 1,800 Calories

Breakfast

Choose one item from row A, one from row B, and two from row C (one with breakfast and one as a mid-morning snack). Choose no more than one item from the column labeled "calorie dense," and only one item from the column labeled "calorie moderate."

	Calorie Light	Calorie Moderate	Calorie Dense
A	• 2 slices French toast with syrup • 3 pancakes with syrup • 2 waffles with syrup • 1 whole plain bagel, any type • 2 plain English muffins • 4 slices plain toast • 2 slices Canadian bacon • 2 egg whites or Egg Beaters	• 1 slice French toast with syrup and butter or margarine • 2 pancakes with syrup and butter or margarine • 1 waffle with syrup and butter or margarine • ½ bagel, any type, with cream cheese • 1 English muffin with butter, margarine, or peanut butter • 1 fried or scrambled egg • 2 slices toast with butter and jelly • 1 sweet roll	• 2 biscuits with butter or margarine • 1 croissant with or without butter or margarine • 1 danish • 1 donut, any type • 1 small slice of quiche
B	• 1 package cream of wheat, instant oatmeal, or other hot cereal	• 2 oz. cold cereal (bran, corn, or wheat flakes, wheat squares, etc.) with 6 oz. skim milk and fruit	• 1 oz. granola-type or sugar-coated cereal with 6 oz. skim milk
C	• 1 piece of fresh fruit (apple, orange, kiwi, grapefruit) • 5 oz. canned fruit in juice or light syrup	• 1 banana • 3 oz. canned fruit in heavy syrup	• 1 oz. coconut, dates, dried fruit, prunes, or raisins

Lunch

Choose one item from row A, one from row B, one from row C, and an afternoon snack from row D. Choose no more than one item from the column labeled "calorie dense," and no more than one item from the column labeled "calorie moderate."

	Calorie Light	Calorie Moderate	Calorie Dense
A	Sandwich with as many vegetables as you want and: • 91% fat-free meat (4 slices) • grilled fish • tuna (in water) • turkey breast • vegetarian	Sandwich with as many vegetables as you want and: • 82–92% fat-free regular lunch meat (2 slices)	• Croissant sandwich with 1 slice low-fat meat • ½ meatball sub • ½ BLT with light mayo • ½ any sandwich with full-fat mayo or cheese • 1 single-patty hamburger
B	• Large garden salad (6 oz.) with no dressing or with fat-free dressing • 8 oz. canned non-cream soup prepared with water	• Medium garden salad (3 oz.) with light salad dressing and croutons or olives • 6 oz. canned cream-type soup prepared with water	• Small garden salad with regular, Caesar, or oil dressing • 4 oz. cream-type soup prepared with skim or low-fat milk
C	8 oz.: • apple juice or cider • grapefruit juice • orange juice • V-8 or tomato juice	5 oz.: • cranberry juice (or other cran-juice) • pineapple juice • prune juice	• 2 oz. coconut milk
D	• 8 oz. nonfat cottage (or other) cheese or low-fat yogurt • 1 Powerbar or Breakbar	• 6 oz. low-fat frozen yogurt • ½ energy bar* • 8 oz. low-fat chocolate milk	• 2–4 oz. any full-fat cheese

* Choose an energy bar that provides a blend of protein, carbohydrates, fat, and fiber (such as Clif Bar, Balance Bar, etc.).

Dinner

Choose one item from row A, one from row B, one from row C, one from row D, and a nighttime snack from row E. Choose no more than one item from the column labeled "calorie dense," and no more than one item from the column labeled "calorie moderate."

	Calorie Light	Calorie Moderate	Calorie Dense
A	• Large garden salad (6 oz.) with no dressing or with fat-free dressing	• Medium garden salad (3 oz.) with light salad dressing and croutons or olives	• Small garden salad with regular, Caesar, or oil dressing
B	6 oz. any 90% fat-free (or better) meat, including: • crab, lobster, shrimp (not fried) • most types broiled fish or other seafood • poultry (white meat, no skin) • 8 oz. beef stew, tuna casserole, or chili	4 oz. any 82% fat-free meat including: • beef flank steak • lean lamb • pork tenderloin • poultry (dark meat, no skin) • regular ham • rveal • 5 oz. macaroni and cheese • 2 slices cheese pizza • 6 oz. pasta with tomato sauce	2.5 oz. any meat less than 82% fat-free, including: • pork chops • beef ribs • fried chicken • fried fish • hotdog, sausage, or kielbasa • poultry with skin • 3 oz. pasta with cream sauce
C	• 2 slices whole-grain bread • 2 whole-grain rolls	• 1 slice whole-grain bread with butter or margarine • 1 croissant	• ½ oz. nuts, seeds, or crackers
D	• Your fill of any vegetable (no butter, margarine, or cheese sauce) • 1 large plain baked or boiled potato • 4 oz. white/brown rice	• 3 oz. rice or potato with butter, margarine, or cheese sauce • 3 oz. flavored rice	• 3 oz. vegetables deep fried or with butter, margarine, or cheese sauce

E
- 1 piece of fresh fruit
- 6 oz. jello
- 2 Popsicles
- 1 low-cal ice cream bar
- ½ cup low-cal pudding

- 4–6 oz. low-fat frozen yogurt
- 1 frozen fudge pop
- ¼ cup regular pudding
- ½ cup sherbet

- 1 oz. (*small* slice) of cake, pie, or pastry
- 1 oz. chocolate
- 1 small scoop low-fat ice cream
- 2 small chocolate-chip cookies
- 3 Fig Newtons

Daily Food-Selection Plan: 2,000 Calories

Breakfast

Choose one item from row A, one from row B, and two from row C (one with breakfast and one as a mid-morning snack). Choose no more than one item from the column labeled "calorie dense," and no more than one item from the column labeled "calorie moderate."

Calorie Light	Calorie Moderate	Calorie Dense
A • 3 slices French toast with syrup • 3–4 pancakes with syrup • 2 Belgian waffles with syrup • 1 whole plain bagel, any type • 2 plain English muffins • 4 slices toast, plain or with jelly • 2–3 slices Canadian bacon • 2–3 egg whites or Egg Beaters	• 1–2 slices French toast with syrup and butter or margarine • 2 pancakes with syrup and butter or margarine • 1 Belgian waffle with syrup and butter or margarine • 1/2 bagel, any type with cream cheese • 1 English muffin with butter, margarine, or peanut butter • 1 fried or scrambled egg • 2 slices toast with butter and jelly • 1 medium sweet roll	• 2 biscuits with butter or margarine • 1 croissant with or without butter or margarine • 1 danish • 1 donut, any type • 1 small slice quiche

B	• 1–2 packages of Cream of Wheat, instant oatmeal, or other hot cereal	• 2–3 oz. cold cereal (bran, corn, or wheat flakes, wheat squares, etc.) with 6 oz. skim milk and fruit	• 1 oz. granola-type or sugar-coated cereal with 6 oz. skim milk
C	• 1–2 pieces of fresh fruit (apple, orange, kiwi, grapefruit) • 5–8 oz. canned fruit in juice or light syrup	• 1–2 medium bananas • 3–5 oz. canned fruit in heavy syrup	• 1–2 oz. coconut, dates, dried fruit, prunes, or raisins

Lunch

Choose one item from row A, one from row B, one from row C, and an afternoon snack from row D. Choose no more than one item from the column labeled "calorie dense," and no more than one item from the column labeled "calorie moderate."

	Calorie Light	Calorie Moderate	Calorie Dense
A	Sandwich with as many vegetables as you want and: • 91% fat-free meat (4–5 slices) • grilled fish • tuna (in water) • turkey breast • vegetarian	Sandwich with as many vegetables as you want and: • 82–92% fat-free regular lunch meat (2–3 slices)	• Croissant sandwich with 1 slice low-fat meat • 1/2 meatball sub • 1/2 BLT with light mayo • 1/2 any sandwich with full-fat mayo or cheese • 1 single-patty hamburger
B	• Large garden salad (6–8 oz.) with no dressing or with fat-free dressing • 8–10 oz. canned noncream soup prepared with water	• Medium garden salad (4 oz.) with light salad dressing and croutons or olives • 6–8 oz. canned cream-type soup prepared with water	• Small garden salad with regular, Caesar, or oil dressing • 4 oz. cream-type soup prepared with skim or low-fat milk

| C | 8–12 oz..
• apple juice or cider
• grapefruit juice
• orange juice
• V-8 or tomato juice | 5–8 oz.:
• cranberry juice (or other cran-juice)
• pineapple juice
• prune juice | • 2–4 oz. coconut milk |
| D | • 8 oz. nonfat cottage (or other) cheese or low-fat yogurt
• 1 Powerbar or Breakbar | • 6 oz. low-fat frozen yogurt
• 1/2 energy bar*
• 8 oz. low-fat chocolate milk | • 2–4 oz. any full-fat cheese |

* Choose an energy bar that provides a blend of protein, carbohydrates, fat, and fiber (such as Clif Bar, Balance Bar, etc.).

Dinner

Choose one item from row A, one from row B, one from row C, one from row D, and a nighttime snack from row E. Choose no more than one item from the column labeled "calorie dense," and no more than one item from the column labeled "calorie moderate."

	Calorie Light	Calorie Moderate	Calorie Dense
A	• Large garden salad (6–8 oz.) with no dressing or with fat-free dressing	• Medium garden salad (4 oz.) with light salad dressing and croutons or olives	• Small garden salad with regular, Caesar, or oil dressing
B	6–8 oz. any 90% fat-free (or better) meat, including: • crab, lobster, shrimp (not fried) • most types broiled fish or other seafood • poultry (white meat, no skin) • 8 oz. beef stew, tuna casserole, or chili	4–6 oz. any 82% fat-free meat, including: • beef flank steak • lean lamb • pork tenderloin • poultry (dark meat, no skin) • regular ham or veal • 5 oz. macaroni and cheese • 2 slices cheese pizza • 6 oz. pasta with tomato sauce	3 oz. any meat less than 82% fat-free including: • pork chops • beef ribs • fried chicken • fried fish • hotdog, sausage, or kielbasa • poultry with skin • 3 oz. pasta with cream sauce

C	• 2–3 slices whole-grain bread • 2–3 whole grain rolls	• 1–2 slices whole-grain bread with butter or margarine • 1 croissant	• ¾ oz. nuts, seeds, or crackers
D	• Your fill of any vegetable (no butter, margarine, or cheese sauce) • 1 large plain baked or boiled potato • 4–6 oz. white/brown rice	• 4 oz. rice or potato with butter, margarine, or cheese sauce • 4 oz. flavored rice	• 3 oz. vegetables deep fried or with butter, margarine, or cheese sauce
E	• 1–2 pieces of fresh fruit • 6 oz. jello • 2 Popsicles • 1–2 low-cal ice cream bars • 1 cup low-cal pudding or yogurt	• 4–6 oz. low-fat frozen yogurt • 1 frozen fudge pop • ½ cup regular pudding • ¾ cup sherbet	• 1–2 oz. (small slice) of cake, pie, or pastry • 1–2 oz. chocolate • 1 small scoop low-fat ice cream • 2 small chocolate-chip cookies • 3 Fig Newtons

References

Chapters 1 to 5

General: Stress, Cortisol Metabolism, and Disease

Abelson, J. L., and G. C. Curtis. "Hypothalamic-Pituitary-Adrenal Axis Activity in Panic Disorder: 24-Hour Secretion of Corticotropin and Cortisol." *Archives of General Psychiatry*, Apr. 1996, 53(4): 323–31.

Al'Alabsi, M., and D. K. Arnett. "Adrenocortical Responses to Psychological Stress and Risk for Hypertension." *Biomedical Pharmacotherapy*, June 2000, 54(5): 234–44.

Andrew, R., D. I. Phillips, and B. R. Walker. "Obesity and Gender Influences on Cortisol Secretion and Metabolism in Man." *Journal of Clinical Endocrinology and Metabolism*, May 1998, 83(5): 1806–9.

Balestreri, R., G. E. Jacopino, E. Foppiani, and N. Elicio. "Aspects of Cortisol Metabolism in Obesity." *Archives of the Maragliano Pathology Clinic*, July–Aug. 1968, 24(4): 431–41.

Balldin, J., K. Blennow, G. Brane, C. G. Gottfries, I. Karlsson, B. Regland, and A. Wallin. "Relationship Between Mental Impairment and HPA Axis Activity in Dementia Disorders." *Dementia*, Sept.–Oct. 1994, 5(5): 252–56.

Biller, B. M., H. J. Federoff, J. I. Koenig, and A. Klibanski. "Abnormal Cortisol Secretion and Responses to Corticotropin-Releasing Hormone in Women with Hypothalamic Amenorrhea." *Journal of Clinical Endocrinology and Metabolism*, Feb. 1990, 70(2): 311–17.

Bjorntorp, P., and R. Rosmond. "Hypothalamic Origin of the Metabolic Syndrome X." *Annual of the New York Academy of Science*, 18 Nov. 1999, 892: 297–307.

Bjorntorp, P., and R. Rosmond. "Obesity and Cortisol." *Nutrition,* Oct. 2000, 16(10): 924–36.

Bjorntorp, P., and R. Rosmond. "The Metabolic Syndrome: A Neuroendocrine Disorder?" *British Journal of Nutrition,* Mar. 2000, 83(suppl. 1): S49–57.

Brillon, D. J., B. Zheng, R. G. Campbell, and D. E. Matthews. "Effect of Cortisol on Energy Expenditure and Amino Acid Metabolism in Humans." *American Journal of Physiology,* 1995, 268: E501–13.

Brindley, D. N. "Neuroendocrine Regulation and Obesity." *International Journal of Obesity and Related Metabolic Disorders,* Dec. 1992, 16(suppl. 3): S73–9.

Catley, D., A. T. Kaell, C. Kirschbaum, and A. A. Stone. "A Naturalistic Evaluation of Cortisol Secretion in Persons with Fibromyalgia and Rheumatoid Arthritis." *Arthritis Care Resources,* Feb. 2000, 13(1): 51–61.

Cauffield, J. S., and H. J. Forbes. "Dietary Supplements Used in the Treatment of Depression, Anxiety, and Sleep Disorders." *Lippincotts Primary Care Practitioner,* May–June 1999, 3(3): 290–304.

Chalew, S., H. Nagel, and S. Shore. "The Hypothalamic-Pituitary-Adrenal Axis in Obesity." *Obesity Resources,* July 1995, 3(4): 371–82.

Chrousos, G. P. "The Role of Stress and the Hypothalamic-Pituitary-Adrenal Axis in the Pathogenesis of the Metabolic Syndrome: Neuro-Endocrine and Target Tissue-Related Causes." *International Journal of Obesity and Related Metabolic Disorders,* June 2000, 24(suppl. 2): S50–55.

Dennison, E., P. Hindmarsh, C. Fall, et al. "Profiles of Endogenous Circulating Cortisol and Bone Mineral Density in Healthy Elderly Men." *Journal of Clinical Endocrinology and Metabolism,* 1999, 84: 3058–63.

Eichner, E. R. "Overtraining: Consequences and Prevention." *Journal of Sports Science,* Summer 1995, 13, spec. no.: S41–48.

Epel, E., R. Lapidus, B. McEwen, and K. Brownell. "Stress May Add Bite to Appetite in Women: A Laboratory Study of Stress-Induced Cortisol and Eating Behavior." *Psychoneuroendocrinology,* 2001, 26: 37–49.

Epel, E. E., A. E. Moyer, C. D. Martin, S. Macary, N. Cummings, J. Rodin, and M. Rebuffe-Scrive. "Stress-Induced Cortisol, Mood, and Fat Distribution in Men." *Obesity Resources,* Oct. 2000, 279(4): R1357–64.

Fry, A. C., W. J. Kraemer, and L. T. Ramsey. "Pituitary-Adrenal-Gonadal Responses to High-Intensity Resistance Exercise Overtraining." *Journal of Applied Physiology,* Dec. 1998, 85(6): 2352–59.

Fry, R. W., J. R. Grove, A. R. Morton, P. M. Zeroni, S. Gaudieri, and D. Keast. "Psychological and Immunological Correlates of Acute Overtraining." *British Journal of Sports Medicine,* Dec. 1994, 28(4): 241–46.

Holmang, A., and P. Bjorntorp. "The Effects of Cortisol on Insulin Sensitivity in Muscle." *Acta Physiologica Scandinavia,* 1992, 144: 425–31.

Jefferies, W. M. "Cortisol and Immunity." *Medical Hypotheses,* Mar. 1991, 34(3): 198–208.

Kelly, G. S. "Nutritional and Botanical Interventions to Assist with the Adaptation to Stress." *Alternative Medicine Review,* Aug. 1999, 4(4): 249–65.

Landsberg, L. "The Sympathoadrenal System, Obesity and Hypertension: An Overview." *Journal of Neuroscience Methods,* Sept. 1990, 34(1-3): 179–86.

Leverenz, J. B., C. W. Wilkinson, M. Wamble, S. Corbin, J. E. Grabber, M. A. Raskind, and E. R. Peskind. "Effect of Chronic High-Dose Exogenous Cortisol on Hippocampal Neuronal Number in Aged Nonhuman Primates." *Journal of Neuroscience,* 15 Mar. 1999, 19(6): 2356–61.

Lewicka, S., M. Nowicki, and P. Vecsei. "Effect of Sodium Restriction on Urinary Excretion of Cortisol and Its Metabolites in Humans." *Steroids,* 1998, 63: 401–5.

Ljung, T., G. Holm, P. Friberg, B. Andersson, B. A. Bengtsson, J. Svensson, M. Dallman, B. McEwen, and P. Bjorntorp. "The Activity of the Hypothalamic-Pituitary-Adrenal Axis and the Sympathetic Nervous System in Relation to Waist/Hip Circumference Ratio in Men." *Obesity Resources,* Oct. 2000, 8(7): 487–95.

Lottenberg, S. A., D. Giannella-Neto, H. Derendorf, et al. "Effect of Fat Distribution on the Pharmacokinetics of Cortisol in Obesity." *International Journal of Clinical Pharmacological Therapy*, 1998, 36: 501–5.

Marin, P., N. Darin, T. Amemiya, B. Andersson, S. Jern, and P. Bjorntorp. "Cortisol Secretion in Relation to Body-Fat Distribution in Obese Premenopausal Women." *Metabolism*, Aug. 1992, 41(8): 882–86.

Matthews, D. E., and A. Battezzati. "Regulation of Protein Metabolism During Stress." *Current Opinions in General Surgery*, 1993: 72–7.

McLean, J. A., S. I. Barr, and J. C. Prior. "Cognitive Dietary Restraint Is Associated with Higher Urinary Cortisol Excretion in Healthy Premenopausal Women." *American Journal of Clinical Nutrition*, 2001, 73: 7–12.

Miller, T. P., J. Taylor, S. Rogerson, M. Mauricio, Q. Kennedy, A. Schatzberg, J. Tinklenberg, and J. Yesavage. "Cognitive and Noncognitive Symptoms in Dementia Patients: Relationship to Cortisol and Dehydroepiandrosterone." *International Psychogeriatrics*, Mar. 1998, 10(1): 85–96.

Mills, F. J. "The Endocrinology of Stress." *Aviation and Space Environmental Medicine*, July 1985, 56(7): 642–50.

Nasman, B., T. Olsson, M. Viitanen, and K. Carlstrom. "A Subtle Disturbance in the Feedback Regulation of the Hypothalamic-Pituitary-Adrenal Axis in the Early Phase of Alzheimer's Disease." *Psychoneuroendocrinology*, 1995, 20(2): 211–20.

Piccirillo, G., F. L. Fimognari, V. Infantino, G. Monteleone, G. B. Fimognari, D. Falletti, and V. Marigliano. "High Plasma Concentrations of Cortisol and Thromboxane B2 in Patients with Depression." *American Journal of Medical Science*, Mar. 1994, 307(3): 228–32.

Pirke, K. M., R. J. Tuschl, B. Spyra, et al. "Endocrine Findings in Restrained Eaters." *Physiology and Behavior*, 1990, 47: 903–6.

Plotsky, P. M., M. J. Owens, and C. B. Nemeroff. "Psychoneuroendocrinology of Depression: Hypothalamic-Pituitary-Adrenal Axis." *Psychiatric Clinics of North America*, June 1998, 21(2): 293–307.

Raber, J. "Detrimental Effects of Chronic Hypothalamic-Pituitary-Adrenal Axis Activation: From Obesity to Memory Deficits." *Molecular Neurobiology*, Aug. 1998, 18(1): 1–22.

Raff, H., J. L. Raff, E. H. Duthie, et al. "Elevated Salivary Cortisol in the Evening in Healthy Elderly Men and Women: Correlation with Bone Mineral Density." *The Journals of Gerontology. Series A, Biological Sciences and Medical Sciences,* 1999, 54: M479–83.

Richdale, A. L., and M. R. Prior. "Urinary Cortisol Circadian Rhythm in a Group of High-Functioning Children with Autism." *Journal of Autism and Developmental Disorders,* Sept. 1992, 22(3): 433–47.

Rosmond, R., and P. Bjorntorp. "Blood Pressure in Relation to Obesity, Insulin and the Hypothalamic-Pituitary-Adrenal Axis in Swedish Men." *Journal of Hypertension,* Dec. 1998, 16(12, pt. 1): 1721–26.

Rosmond, R., and P. Bjorntorp. "Occupational Status, Cortisol Secretory Pattern, and Visceral Obesity in Middle-Aged Men." *Obesity Resources,* Sept. 2000, 8(6): 445–50.

Rosmond, R., M. F. Dallman, and P. Bjorntorp. "Stress-Related Cortisol Secretion in Men: Relationships with Abdominal Obesity and Endocrine, Metabolic and Hemodynamic Abnormalities." *Journal of Clinical Endocrinology and Metabolism,* June 1998, 83(6): 1853–59.

Rosmond, R., G. Holm, and P. Bjorntorp. "Food-Induced Cortisol Secretion in Relation to Anthropometric, Metabolic and Haemodynamic Variables in Men." *International Journal of Obesity and Related Metabolic Disorders,* 2000, 24: 416–22.

Sapolsky, R. M., and P. M. Plotsky. "Hypercortisolism and Its Possible Neural Bases." *Biological Psychiatry,* 1 May 1990, 27(9): 937–52.

Sapse, A. T. "Cortisol, High-Cortisol Diseases and Anti-Cortisol Therapy." *Psychoneuroendocrinology,* 1997, 22(suppl. 1): S3–10.

Svec, F., and A. L. Shawar. "The Acute Effect of a Noontime Meal on the Serum Levels of Cortisol and DHEA in Lean and Obese Women." *Psychoneuroendocrinology,* 1997, 22(suppl. 1): S115–19.

Swaab, D. F., F. C. Raadsheer, E. Endert, M. A. Hofman, W. Kamphorst, and R. Ravid. "Increased Cortisol Levels in Aging and Alzheimer's Disease in Postmortem Cerebrospinal Fluid." *Journal of Neuroendocrinology,* Dec. 1994, 6(6): 681–87.

Takahara, J., H. Hosogi, S. Yunoki, K. Hashimoto, and T. Uneki. "Hypothalamic Pituitary Adrenal Function in Patients with Anorexia Nervosa." *Endocrinology-Japan,* Dec. 1976, 23(6): 451–56.

Tsigos, C., R. J. Young, and A. White. "Diabetic Neuropathy Is Associated with Increased Activity of the Hypothalamic-Pituitary-Adrenal Axis." *Journal of Clinical Endocrinology and Metabolism*, Mar. 1993, 76(3): 554–58.

Varma, V. K., J. T. Rushing, and W. H. Ettinger, Jr. "High Density Lipoprotein Cholesterol Is Associated with Serum Cortisol in Older People." *Journal of the American Geriatric Society*, 1995, 43: 1345–59.

Vicennati, V., and R. Pasquali. "Abnormalities of the Hypothalamic-Pituitary-Adrenal Axis in Nondepressed Women with Abdominal Obesity and Relations with Insulin Resistance: Evidence for a Central and a Peripheral Alteration." *Journal of Clinical Endocrinology and Metabolism*, Nov. 2000, 85(11): 4093–98.

Walder, D. J., E. F. Walker, and R. J. Lewine. "Cognitive Functioning, Cortisol Release, and Symptom Severity in Patients with Schizophrenia." *Biological Psychiatry*, 15 Dec. 2000, 48(12): 1121–32.

Walker, B. R., S. Soderberg, B. Lindahl, and T. Olsson. "Independent Effects of Obesity and Cortisol in Predicting Cardiovascular Risk Factors in Men and Women." *Journal of Internal Medicine*, Feb. 2000, 247(2): 198–204.

Weiner, M. F., S. Vobach, D. Svetlik, and R. C. Risser. "Cortisol Secretion and Alzheimer's Disease Progression: A Preliminary Report." *Biological Psychiatry*, 1 Aug. 1993, 34(3): 158–61.

Chapter 6: Dietary Supplements to Avoid

General: Cortisol and Herbal Stimulants

Al'Absi, M., W. R. Lovallo, B. McKey, B. H. Sung, T. L. Whitsett, and M. F. Wilson. "Hypothalamic-Pituitary-Adrenocortical Responses to Psychological Stress and Caffeine in Men at High and Low Risk for Hypertension." *Psychosomatic Medicine*, July–Aug. 1998, 60(4): 521–27.

Charney, D. S., G. R. Heninger, and P. I. Jatlow. "Increased Anxiogenic Effects of Caffeine in Panic Disorders." *Archives of General Psychiatry*, Mar. 1985, 42(3): 233–43.

Gilbert, D. G., W. D. Dibb, L. C. Plath, and S. G. Hiyane. "Effects of Nicotine and Caffeine, Separately and in Combination, on EEG Topography, Mood, Heart Rate, Cortisol, and Vigilance." *Psychophysiology*, Sept. 2000, 37(5): 583–95.

Lovallo, W. R., M. al'Absi, K. Blick, T. L. Whitsett, and M. F. Wilson. "Stress-Like Adrenocorticotropin Responses to Caffeine in Young Healthy Men." *Pharmacology, Biochemistry, and Behavior,* Nov. 1996, 55(3): 365–69.

Lovallo, W. R., G. A. Pincomb, B. H. Sung, R. B. Passey, K. P. Sausen, and M. F. Wilson. "Caffeine May Potentiate Adrenocortical Stress Responses in Hypertension-Prone Men." *Hypertension,* Aug. 1989, 14(2): 170–76.

Mattila, M., T. Seppala, and M. J. Mattila. "Anxiogenic Effect of Yohimbine in Healthy Subjects: Comparison with Caffeine and Antagonism by Clonidine and Diazepam." *International Clinical Psychopharmacology,* July 1988, 3(3): 215–29.

Paquot, N., P. Schneiter, E. Jequier, and L. Tappy. "Effects of Glucocorticoids and Sympathomimetic Agents on Basal and Insulin-Stimulated Glucose Metabolism." *Clinical Physiology,* May 1995, 15(3): 231–40.

Pincomb, G. A., W. R. Lovallo, R. B. Passey, D. J. Brackett, and M. F. Wilson. "Caffeine Enhances the Physiological Response to Occupational Stress in Medical Students." *Health and Psychology,* 1987, 6(2): 101–12.

Shepard, J. D., M. al'Absi, T. L. Whitsett, R. B. Passey, and W. R. Lovallo. "Additive Pressor Effects of Caffeine and Stress in Male Medical Students at Risk for Hypertension." *American Journal of Hypertension,* May 2000, 13(5, pt. 1): 475–81.

Ephedra/Ma Huang/Sida Cordifolia

Astrup, A., et al. "The Effect and Safety of an Ephedrine/Caffeine Compound Compared to Ephedrine, Caffeine and Placebo in Obese Subjects on an Energy-Restricted Diet: A Double-Blind Trial." *International Journal of Obesity and Related Metabolic Disorders,* 1992, 16(4): 269–77.

Astrup, A., L. Breum, and S. Toubro. "Pharmacological and Clinical Studies of Ephedrine and Other Thermogenic Agonists." *Obesity Research,* 1995, 3(suppl. 4): S537–40.

Breum, L., et al. "Comparison of an Ephedrine/Caffeine Combination and Dexfenfluramine in the Treatment of Obesity: A Double-Blind Multi-Centre Trial in General Practice." *International Journal of Obesity and Related Metabolic Disorders,* 1994, 18(2): 99–103.

Daly, P. A., et al. "Ephedrine, Caffeine and Aspirin: Safety and Efficacy for Treatment of Human Obesity." *International Journal of Obesity and Related Metabolic Disorders*, 1993, 17(suppl. 1): S73-78.

Gurley, B. J., S. F. Gardner, and M. A. Hubbard. "Content Versus Label Claims in Ephedra-Containing Dietary Supplements." *American Journal of Health Systems Pharmacology*, 15 May 2000, 57(10): 963–69.

Toubro, S., et al. "Safety and Efficacy of Long-Term Treatment with Ephedrine, Caffeine and an Ephedrine/Caffeine Mixture." *International Journal of Obesity and Related Metabolic Disorders*, 1993, 17(suppl. 1): S69–72.

Toubro, S., et al. "The Acute and Chronic Effects of Ephedrine/Caffeine Mixtures on Energy Expenditure and Glucose Metabolism in Humans." *International Journal of Obesity and Related Metabolic Disorders*, 1993, 17(suppl. 3): S73–77; discussion S82.

Guarana

Galduroz, J. C., and E. de A. Carlini. "Acute Effects of the Paullinia Cupana 'Guarana' on the Cognition of Normal Volunteers." *Revista Paulista de Medicina*, July–Sept. 1994, 112(3): 607–11.

Galduroz, J. C., and E. de A. Carlini. "The Effects of Long-Term Administration of Guarana on the Cognition of Normal, Elderly Volunteers." *Revista Paulista de Medicina*, Jan.–Feb. 1996, 114(1): 1073–78.

Katzung, W. "Guarana: A Natural Product with High Caffeine Content." *Medizinische Monatsschrift Pharmazeuten*, Nov. 1993, 16(11): 330–33.

Synephrine/Zhi Shi/Citrus Aurantium

Chen, X., L. Y. Liu, H. W. Deng, Y. X. Fang, and Y. W. Ye. "The Effects of Citrus Aurantium and Its Active Ingredient N-Methyltyramine on the Cardiovascular Receptors." *Yao Hsueh Hsueh Pao*, Apr. 1981, 16(4): 253–59.

Fontana, E., N. Morin, D. Prevot, and C. Carpene. "Effects of Octopamine on Lipolysis, Glucose Transport and Amine Oxidation in Mammalian Fat Cells." *Comparative Biochemistry and Physiology. C, Comparative Pharmacology, Toxicology, and Endocrinology*, Jan. 2000, 125(1): 33–44.

Galitzky, J., C. Carpene, M. Lafontan, and M. Berlan. "Specific Stimulation of Adipose Tissue Adrenergic Beta 3 Receptors by Octopamine." *Comptes Rendus de l'Academie des Sciences. Serie III, Sciences de la Vie,* 1993, 316(5): 519–23.

Penzak, S. R., et al. "Seville (sour) orange juice: synephrine content and cardiovascular effects in normotensive adults." *Journal of Clinical Pharmacology,* Oct. 2001, 41(10): 1059–63.

Preuss, H. G., et al. "Citrus aurantium as a therapeutic, weight-reduction replacement for ephedra: an overview." *Journal of Medicine,* 2002, 33(1–4): 247–64.

Yohimbe/Quebracho

Adimoelja, A. "Phytochemicals and the Breakthrough of Traditional Herbs in the Management of Sexual Dysfunctions." *International Journal of Andrology,* 2000, 23(suppl. 2): 82–84.

De Smet, P. A., and O. S. Smeets. "Potential Risks of Health-Food Products Containing Yohimbe Extracts." *British Medical Journal,* 8 Oct. 1994, 309(6959): 958.

Coleus

Greenway, F. L., and G. A. Bray. "Regional Fat Loss from the Thigh in Obese Women after Adrenergic Modulation." *Clinical Therapy,* 1987, 9(6): 663–69.

Martin, L. F., C. M. Klim, S. J. Vannucci, L. B. Dixon, J. R. Landis, and K. F. LaNoue. "Alterations in Adipocyte Adenylate Cyclase Activity in Morbidly Obese and Formerly Morbidly Obese Humans." *Surgery,* Aug. 1990, 108(2): 228–34; discussion 234–35.

Mauriege, P., D. Prud'homme, S. Lemieux, A. Tremblay, and J. P. Despres. "Regional Differences in Adipose Tissue Lipolysis from Lean and Obese Women: Existence of Postreceptor Alterations." *American Journal of Physiology,* Aug. 1995, 269(2, pt. 1): E341–50.

Mauriege, P., D. Prud'homme, M. Marcotte, M. Yoshioka, A. Tremblay, and J. P. Despres. "Regional Differences in Adipose Tissue Metabolism Between Sedentary and Endurance-Trained Women." *American Journal of Physiology,* Sept. 1997, 273(3, pt. 1): E497–506.

Van Belle, H. "Is There a Role for cAMP and Adenyl Cyclase?" *Journal of Cardiovascular Pharmacology,* 1985, 7(suppl. 5): S28–32.

Chapter 7: Vitamins and Minerals for Stress Adaptation

Vitamin C

Halliwell, B. "Antioxidant Defence Mechanisms: From the Beginning to the End (of the Beginning)." *Free-Radical Research,* Oct. 1999, 31(4): 261–72.

Jacob, R. A., F. S. Pianalto, and R. E. Agee. "Cellular Ascorbate Depletion in Healthy Men." *Journal of Nutrition,* May 1992, 122(5): 1111–18.

Johnston, C. S., C. G. Meyer, and J. C. Srilakshmi. "Vitamin C Elevates Red Blood Cell Glutathione in Healthy Adults." *American Journal of Clinical Nutrition,* July 1993, 58(1): 103–5.

Rokitzki, L., S. Hinkel, C. Klemp, D. Cufi, and J. Keul. "Dietary, Serum and Urine Ascorbic Acid Status in Male Athletes." *International Journal of Sports Medicine,* Oct. 1994, 15(7): 435–40.

Sinclair, A. J., P. B. Taylor, J. Lunec, A. J. Girling, and A. H. Barnett. "Low Plasma Ascorbate Levels in Patients with Type-2 Diabetes Mellitus Consuming Adequate Dietary Vitamin C." *Diabetes Medicine,* Nov. 1994, 11(9): 893–98.

VanderJagt, D. J., P. J. Garry, and H. N. Bhagavan. "Ascorbic Acid Intake and Plasma Levels in Healthy Elderly People." *American Journal of Clinical Nutrition,* Aug. 1987, 46(2): 290–94.

Magnesium

Altura, B. M., and B. T. Altura. "New Perspectives on the Role of Magnesium in the Pathophysiology of the Cardiovascular System: Clinical Aspects." *Magnesium,* 1985, 4(5-6): 226–44.

Paddle, B. M., and N. Haugaard. "Role of Magnesium in Effects of Epinephrine on Heart Contraction and Metabolism." *American Journal of Physiology,* Oct. 1971, 221(4): 1178–84.

Savabi, F., V. Gura, S. Bessman, and N. Brautbar. "Effects of Magnesium Depletion on Myocardial High-Energy Phosphates and Contractility." *Biochemical Medicine and Metabolic Biology,* Apr. 1988, 39(2): 131–39.

Zimmermann, P., U. Weiss, H. G. Classen, B. Wendt, A. Epple, H. Zollner, W. Temmel, M. Weger, and S. Porta. "The Impact of Diets with

Different Magnesium Contents on Magnesium and Calcium in Serum and Tissues of the Rat." *Life Sciences,* 14 July 2000, 67(8): 949–58.

B-Complex Vitamins (Thiamin, Riboflavin, Pantothenic Acid, Pyridoxine)

Baldewicz, T., K. Goodkin, D. J. Feaster, N. T. Blaney, M. Kumar, A. Kumar, G. Shor-Posner, and M. Baum. "Plasma Pyridoxine Deficiency Is Related to Increased Psychological Distress in Recently Bereaved Homosexual Men." *Psychosomatic Medicine,* May–June 1998, 60(3): 297–308.

Bendich, A. "The Potential for Dietary Supplements to Reduce Premenstrual Syndrome (PMS) Symptoms." *Journal of the American College of Nutrition,* Feb. 2000, 19(1): 3–12.

Bigazzi, M., S. Ferraro, R. Ronga, G. Scarselli, V. Bruni, and A. L. Olivotti. "Effect of Vitamin B-6 on the Serum Concentration of Pituitary Hormones in Normal Humans and under Pathologic Conditions." *Journal of Endocrinological Investigation,* Apr.–June 1979, 2(2): 117–24.

Heap, L. C., T. J. Peters, and S. Wessely. "Vitamin B Status in Patients with Chronic Fatigue Syndrome." *Journal of the Royal Society of Medicine,* Apr. 1999, 92(4): 183–85.

Kopp-Woodroffe, S. A., M. M. Manore, C. A. Dueck, J. S. Skinner, and K. S. Matt. "Energy and Nutrient Status of Amenorrheic Athletes Participating in a Diet and Exercise Training Intervention Program." *International Journal of Sport Nutrition,* Mar. 1999, 9(1): 70–88.

Leung, L. H. "Pantothenic Acid as a Weight-Reducing Agent: Fasting Without Hunger, Weakness and Ketosis." *Medical Hypotheses,* May 1995, 44(5): 403–5.

Manore, M. M. "Effect of Physical Activity on Thiamine, Riboflavin, and Vitamin B-6 Requirements." *American Journal of Clinical Nutrition,* Aug. 2000, 72(2, suppl.): S598–606.

Chapter 8: Cortisol-Control Supplements

Magnolia Bark

Kuribara, H., et al. "The Anxiolytic Effect of Two Oriental Herbal Drugs in Japan Attributed to Honokiol from Magnolia Bark." *Journal of Pharmacy and Pharmacology,* 2000, 52(11): 1425–29.

Wang, S. M., et al. "Magnolol Stimulates Steroidogenesis in Rat Adrenal Cells." *British Journal of Pharmacology*, 2000, 131(6): 1172–78.

Watanabe, K., Y. Goto, and K. Yoshitomi. "Central Depressant Effects of the Extracts of Magnolia Cortex." *Chemical and Pharmacological Bulletin.* Tokyo, 1973, 21: 1700–8.

Watanabe, K., H. Watanabe, Y. Goto, M. Yamaguchi, N. Yamamoto, and K. Hagino. "Pharmacological Properties of Magnolol and Honokiol Extracted from Magnolia Officinalis: Central Depressant Effects." *Planta Medica*, 1983, 49: 103–8.

Watanabe, K., H. Y. Watanabe, Y. Goto, N. Yamamoto, and M. Yoshizaki. "Studies on the Active Principles of Magnolia Bark: Centrally Acting Muscle Relaxant Activity of Magnolol and Honokiol." *Japanese Journal of Pharmacology*, 1975, 25: 605–7.

Theanine

Kakuda, T., A. Nozawa, T. Unno, N. Okamura, and O. Okai. "Inhibiting Effects of Theanine on Caffeine Stimulation Evaluated by EEG in the Rat." *Biosciences, Biotechnology, and Biochemistry*, Feb. 2000, 64(2): 287–93.

Yokogoshi, H., Y. Kato, Y. M. Sagesaka, T. Takihara-Matsuura, T. Kakuda, and N. Takeuchi. "Reduction Effect of Theanine on Blood Pressure and Brain 5-Hydroxyindoles in Spontaneously Hypertensive Rats." *Biosciences, Biotechnology, and Biochemistry*, Apr. 1995, 59(4): 615–18.

Yokogoshi, H., T. Terashima. "Effect of Theanine, R-Glutamylethylamide, on Brain Monoamines, Striatal Dopamine Release and Some Kinds of Behavior in Rats." *Nutrition*, Sept. 2000, 16(9): 776–77.

Epimedium

Cai, D., S. Shen, and X. Chen. "Clinical and Experimental Research of Epimedium Brevicornum in Relieving Neuroendocrino-Immunological Effect Inhibited by Exogenous Glucocorticoid." *Zhongguo Zhong Xi Yi Jie He Za Zhi*, Jan. 1998, 18(1): 4–7.

Kuang, A. K., J. L. Chen, and M. D. Chen. "Effects of Yang-Restoring Herb Medicines on the Levels of Plasma Corticosterone, Testosterone and Triiodothyronine." *Zhong Xi Yi Jie He Za Zhi*, Dec. 1989, 9(12): 737–38, 710.

Zhang, J. Q. "Clinical and Experimental Studies on Yang Deficiency." *Journal of Traditional Chinese Medicine*, Sept. 1982, 2(3): 237–42.

Zhong, L. Y., Z. Y. Shen, and D. F. Cai. "Effect of Three Kinds (Tonifying Kidney, Invigorating Spleen, Promoting Blood Circulation) Recipes on the Hypothalamus-Pituitary-Adrenal-Thymus (HPAT) Axis and CRF Gene Expression." *Zhongguo Zhong Xi Yi Jie He Za Zhi*, Jan. 1997, 17(1): 39–41.

Phytosterols

Agren, J. J., E. Tvrzicka, M. T. Nenonen, T. Helve, and O. Hanninen. "Divergent Changes in Serum Sterols During a Strict Uncooked Vegan Diet in Patients with Rheumatoid Arthritis." *British Journal of Nutrition*, Feb. 2001, 85(2): 137–39.

Bouic, P. J., and J. H. Lamprecht. "Plant Sterols and Sterolins: A Review of Their Immune-Modulating Properties." *Alternative Medicine Review*, June 1999, 4(3): 170–77.

"Plant Sterols and Sterolins." *Alternative Medicine Review*, Apr. 2001, 6(2): 203–6.

Phosphatidylserine

Diboune, M., G. Ferard, Y. Ingenbleek, A. Bourguignat, D. Spielmann, C. Scheppler-Roupert, P. A. Tulasne, B. Calon, M. Hasselmann, P. Sauder, et al. "Soybean Oil, Blackcurrant Seed Oil, Medium-Chain Triglycerides, and Plasma Phospholipid Fatty Acids of Stressed Patients." *Nutrition*, July–Aug. 1993, 9(4): 344–49.

Leathwood, P. D. "Neurotransmitter Precursors and Brain Function." *Bibliotheca Nutritio et Dieta*, 1986, (38): 54–71.

Monteleone, P., L. Beinat, C. Tanzillo, M. Maj, and D. Kemali. "Effects of Phosphatidylserine on the Neuroendocrine Response to Physical Stress in Humans." *Neuroendocrinology*, Sept. 1990, 52(3): 243–58.

Monteleone, P., M. Maj, L. Beinat, M. Natale, and D. Kemali. "Blunting by Chronic Phosphatidylserine Administration of the Stress-Induced Activation of the Hypothalamo-Pituitary-Adrenal Axis in Healthy Men." *European Journal of Clinical Pharmacology*, 1992, 42(4): 385–88.

Wurtman, R. J. "Nutrients That Modify Brain Function." *Scientific American*, Apr. 1982, 246(4): 50–9.

Tyrosine

Acworth, I. N., M. J. During, and R. J. Wurtman. "Tyrosine: Effects on Catecholamine Release." *Brain Research Bulletin*, Sept. 1988, 21(3): 473–77.

Caballero, B., R. E. Gleason, and R. J. Wurtman. "Plasma Amino Acid Concentrations in Healthy Elderly Men and Women." *American Journal of Clinical Nutrition*, May 1991, 53(5): 1249–52.

Conlay, L. A., R. J. Wurtman, G. Lopez, I. Coviella, J. K. Blusztajn, C. A. Vacanti, M. Logue, M. During, B. Caballero, T. J. Maher, and G. Evoniuk. "Effects of Running the Boston Marathon on Plasma Concentrations of Large Neutral Amino Acids." *Journal of Neural Transmission*, 1989, 76(1): 65–71.

Dollins, A. B., L. P. Krock, W. F. Storm, R. J. Wurtman, and H. R. Lieberman. "L-Tyrosine Ameliorates Some Effects of Lower Body Negative Pressure Stress." *Physiology and Behavior*, Feb. 1995, 57(2): 223–30.

Lieberman, H. R., S. Corkin, B. J. Spring, R. J. Wurtman, and J. H. Growdon. "The Effects of Dietary Neurotransmitter Precursors on Human Behavior." *American Journal of Clinical Nutrition*, Aug. 1985, 42(2): 366–70.

Milner, J. D., and R. J. Wurtman. "Tyrosine Availability: A Presynaptic Factor Controlling Catecholamine Release." *Advances in Experimental Medicine and Biology*, 1987, 221: 211–21.

Reinstein, D. K., H. Lehnert, and R. J. Wurtman. "Dietary Tyrosine Suppresses the Rise in Plasma Corticosterone Following Acute Stress in Rats." *Life Sciences*, 9 Dec. 1985, 37(23): 2157–63.

Wurtman, R. J. "Effects of Their Nutrient Precursors on the Synthesis and Release of Serotonin, the Catecholamines, and Acetylcholine: Implications for Behavioral Disorders." *Clinical Neuropharmacology*, 1988, 11(suppl. 1): S187–93.

Branched-Chain Amino Acids (BCAAs; Valine, Leucine, and Isoleucine)

Blomstrand, E., F. Celsing, and E. A. Newsholme. "Changes in Plasma Concentrations of Aromatic and Branched-Chain Amino Acids During

Sustained Exercise in Man and Their Possible Role in Fatigue." *Acta Physiologica Scandinavia,* May 1988, 133(1): 115–21.

Blomstrand, E., P. Hassmen, S. Ek, B. Ekblom, and E. A. Newsholme. "Influence of Ingesting a Solution of Branched-Chain Amino Acids on Perceived Exertion During Exercise." *Acta Physiologica Scandinavia,* Jan. 1997, 159(1): 41–49.

Castell, L. M., T. Yamamoto, J. Phoenix, and E. A. Newsholme. "The Role of Tryptophan in Fatigue in Different Conditions of Stress." *Advances in Experimental Medicine and Biology,* 1999, 467: 697–704.

Davis, J. M., R. S. Welsh, K. L. De Volve, and N. A. Alderson. "Effects of Branched-Chain Amino Acids and Carbohydrate on Fatigue During Intermittent, High-Intensity Running." *International Journal of Sports Medicine,* July 1999, 20(5): 309–14.

Gastmann, U. A., and M. J. Lehmann. "Overtraining and the BCAA Hypothesis." *Medicine and Science in Sports and Exercise,* July 1998, 30(7): 1173–78.

Hassmen, P., E. Blomstrand, B. Ekblom, and E. A. Newsholme. "Branched-Chain Amino Acid Supplementation During 30-Km Competitive Run: Mood and Cognitive Performance." *Nutrition,* Sept.–Oct. 1994, 10(5): 405–10.

Lehmann, M., M. Huonker, F. Dimeo, N. Heinz, U. Gastmann, N. Treis, J. M. Steinacker, J. Keul, R. Kajewski, and D. Haussinger. "Serum Amino Acid Concentrations in Nine Athletes Before and After the 1993 Colmar Ultra Triathlon." *International Journal of Sports Medicine,* Apr. 1995, 16(3): 155–69.

Mittleman, K. D., M. R. Ricci, S. P. Bailey. "Branched-Chain Amino Acids Prolong Exercise During Heat Stress in Men and Women." *Medicine and Science in Sports and Exercise,* Jan. 1998, 30(1): 83–91.

Chapter 9: Adaptogens (General Antistress Supplements)

Ginseng

Avakian, E. V., R. B. Sugimoto, S. Taguchi, and S. M. Horvath. "Effect of Panax Ginseng Extract on Energy Metabolism During Exercise in Rats." *Planta Medica,* Apr. 1984, 50(2): 151–54.

Dowling, E. A., D. R. Redondo, J. D. Branch, S. Jones, G. McNabb, and M. H. Williams. "Effect of Eleutherococcus Senticosus on Submaximal and Maximal Exercise Performance." *Medical Science, Sports, and Exercise,* Apr. 1996, 28(4): 482–89.

Wang, B. X., J. C. Cui, A. J. Liu, and S. K. Wu. "Studies on the Anti-Fatigue Effect of the Saponins of Stems and Leaves of Panax Ginseng (SSLG)." *Journal of Traditional Chinese Medicine,* June 1983, 3(2): 89–94.

Wang, L. C., and T. F. Lee. "Effect of Ginseng Saponins on Exercise Performance in Non-Trained Rats." *Planta Medica,* Mar. 1998, 64(2): 130–33.

Ziemba, A. W., J. Chmura, H. Kaciuba-Uscilko, K. Nazar, P. Wisnik, and W. Gawronski. "Ginseng Treatment Improves Psychomotor Performance at Rest and During Graded Exercise in Young Athletes." *International Journal of Sport Nutrition,* Dec. 1999, 9(4): 371–77.

Ashwagandha

Bhattacharya, S. K., A. Bhattacharya, K. Sairam, and S. Ghosal. "Anxiolytic-Antidepressant Activity of Withania Somnifera Glycowithanolides: An Experimental Study." *Phytomedicine,* Dec. 2000, 7(6): 463–69.

Dhuley, J. N. "Adaptogenic and Cardioprotective Action of Ashwagandha in Rats and Frogs." *Journal of Ethnopharmacology,* Apr. 2000, 70(1): 57–63.

Dhuley, J. N. "Effect of Ashwagandha on Lipid Peroxidation in Stress-Induced Animals." *Journal of Ethnopharmacology,* Mar. 1998, 60(2): 173–78.

Mishra, L. C., B. B. Singh, and S. Dagenais. "Scientific Basis for the Therapeutic Use of Withania Somnifera (Ashwagandha): A Review." *Alternative Medicine Review,* Aug. 2000, 5(4): 334–46.

Ziauddin, M., N. Phansalkar, P. Patki, S. Diwanay, and B. Patwardhan. "Studies on the Immunomodulatory Effects of Ashwagandha." *Journal of Ethnopharmacology,* Feb. 1996, 50(2): 69–76.

Suma

Arletti, R., A. Benelli, E. Cavazzuri, G. Scarpetta, and A. Bertolini. "Stimulating Property of Turnera Diffusa and Pfaffia Paniculata Extracts on the Sexual Behavior of Male Rats." *Psychopharmacology.* Berlin, Mar. 1999, 143(1): 15–19.

Watanabe, T., M. Watanabe, Y. Watanabe, and C. Hotta. "Effects of Oral Administration of Pfaffia Paniculata (Brazilian Ginseng) on Incidence of Spontaneous Leukemia in AKR/J Mice." *Cancer Detection and Prevention,* 2000, 24(2): 173–78.

Schisandra

Li, P. C., K. T. Poon, and K. M. Ko. "Schisandra Chinensis-Dependent Myocardial Protective Action of Sheng-Mai-San in Rats." *American Journal of Chinese Medicine,* 1996, 24(3-4): 255–62.

Liu, G. T. "Advances in Research of the Action of Components Isolated from Fructus Schizandrae Chinensis on Animal Livers." *Chung Hsi I Chieh Ho Tsa Chih,* May 1983, 3(3): 182–85.

Yan-yong, C., S. Zeng-bao, and L. Lian-niang. "Studies of Fructus Schizandrae IV: Isolation and Determination of the Active Compounds (in Lowering High SGPT Levels) of Schizandra Chinensis." *Baillieres Scientifica Sinica.* Mar.–Apr. 1976, 19(2): 276–90.

Rhodiola

Maslova, L. V., B. Iu. Kondrat'ev, L. N. Maslov, and Iu. B. Lishmanov. "The Cardioprotective and Antiadrenergic Activity of an Extract of Rhodiola Rosea in Stress." *Eksperimental Klinicheskaia Farmakologiia,* Nov.–Dec. 1994, 57(6): 61–63.

Rege, N. N., U. M. Thatte, and S. A. Dahanukar. "Adaptogenic Properties of Six Rasayana Herbs Used in Ayurvedic Medicine." *Phytotherapy Research,* June 1999, 13(4): 275–91.

Spasov, A. A., G. K. Wikman, V. B. Mandrikov, I. A. Mironova, and V. V. Neumoin. "A Double-Blind, Placebo-Controlled Pilot Study of the Stimulating and Adaptogenic Effect of Rhodiola Rosea SHR-5 Extract on the Fatigue of Students Caused by Stress During an Examination Period with a Repeated Low-Dose Regimen." *Phytomedicine,* Apr. 2000, 7(2): 85–89.

Astragalus

Sinclair, S. "Chinese Herbs: A Clinical Review of Astragalus, Ligusticum, and Schizandrae." *Alternative Medicine Review,* Oct. 1998, 3(5): 338–44.

Sugiura, H., H. Nishida, R. Inaba, and H. Iwata. "Effects of Exercise in the Growing Stage in Mice and of Astragalus Membranaceus on Immune Functions." *Nippon Eiseigaku Zasshi,* Feb. 1993, 47(6): 1021–31.

Sun, Y., E. M. Hersh, M. Talpaz, S. L. Lee, W. Wong, T. L. Loo, and G. M. Mavligit. "Immune Restoration and/or Augmentation of Local Graft Versus Host Reaction by Traditional Chinese Medicinal Herbs." *Cancer,* 1 July 1983, 52(1): 70–73.

Zhao, K. S., C. Mancini, and G. Doria. "Enhancement of the Immune Response in Mice by Astragalus Membranaceus Extracts." *Immunopharmacology,* Nov.–Dec. 1990, 20(3): 225–33.

Chapter 10: Relaxation and Calming Supplements

Kava Kava

Heiligenstein, E., and G. Guenther. "Over-the-Counter Psychotropics: A Review of Melatonin, St. John's Wort, Valerian, and Kava-Kava." *Journal of the American College of Health,* May 1998, 46(6): 271–76.

Herberg, K. W. "Effect of Kava-Special Extract WS 1490 Combined with Ethyl Alcohol on Safety-Relevant Performance Parameters." *Blutalkohol,* Mar. 1993, 30(2): 96–105.

Muller, B., and R. Komorek. "Treatment with Kava: The Root to Combat Stress." *Wiener Medzinische Wochenschrift,* 1999, 149(8–10): 197–201.

Pittler, M. H., and E. Ernst. "Efficacy of Kava Extract for Treating Anxiety: Systematic Review and Meta-Analysis." *Journal of Clinical Psychopharmacology,* Feb. 2000, 20(1): 84–89.

Scherer, J. "Kava-Kava Extract in Anxiety Disorders: An Outpatient Observational Study." *Advances in Therapy.* July–Aug. 1998, 15(4): 261–69.

Volz, H. P., and M. Kieser. "Kava-Kava Extract WS 1490 Versus Placebo in Anxiety Disorders: A Randomized Placebo-Controlled 25-Week Outpatient Trial." *Pharmacopsychiatry*, Jan. 1997, 30(1): 1–5.

Melatonin

Arendt, J., and S. Deacon. "Treatment of Circadian Rhythm Disorders: Melatonin." *Chronobiology International*, Mar. 1997, 14(2): 185–204.

Chase, J. E., and B. E. Gidal. "Melatonin: Therapeutic Use in Sleep Disorders." *Annals of Pharmacotherapy*, Oct. 1997, 31(10): 1218–26.

Defrance, R., and M. A. Quera-Salva. "Therapeutic Applications of Melatonin and Related Compounds." *Hormone Research*, 1998, 49(3-4): 142–46.

Jan, J. E., H. Espezel, R. D. Freeman, and D. K. Fast. "Melatonin Treatment of Chronic Sleep Disorders." *Journal of Childhood Neurology*, Feb. 1998, 13(2): 98.

Okawa, M., M. Uchiyama, S. Ozaki, K. Shibui, Y. Kamei, T. Hayakawa, and J. Urata. "Melatonin Treatment for Circadian Rhythm Sleep Disorders." *Psychiatry and Clinical Neuroscience*, Apr. 1998, 52(2): 259–60.

Sack, R. L., R. J. Hughes, D. M. Edgar, and A. J. Lewy. "Sleep-Promoting Effects of Melatonin: At What Dose, in Whom, under What Conditions, and by What Mechanisms?" *Sleep*, Oct. 1997, 20(10): 908–15.

Sack, R. L., A. J. Lewy, and R. J. Hughes. "Use of Melatonin for Sleep and Circadian Rhythm Disorders." *Annals of Medicine*, Feb. 1998, 30(1): 115–21.

Valerian

Balderer, G., and A. A. Borbely. "Effect of Valerian on Human Sleep." *Psychopharmacology*, Berlin, 1985, 87(4): 406–9.

Donath, F., S. Quispe, K. Diefenbach, A. Maurer, I. Fietze, and I. Roots. "Critical Evaluation of the Effect of Valerian Extract on Sleep Structure and Sleep Quality." *Pharmacopsychiatry*, Mar. 2000, 33(2): 47–53.

Houghton, P. J. "The Biological Activity of Valerian and Related Plants." *Journal of Ethnopharmacology*, Feb.–Mar., 1988, 22(2): 121–42.

Schmitz, M., and M. Jackel. "Comparative Study for Assessing Quality of Life of Patients with Exogenous Sleep Disorders (Temporary Sleep Onset and Sleep Interruption Disorders) Treated with a Hops-Valerian Preparation and a Benzodiazepine Drug." *Wiener Medizinische Wochenschrift,* 1998, 148(13): 291–98.

Gotu Kola

Bradwejn, J., Y. Zhou, D. Koszycki, J. Shlik. "A Double-Blind, Placebo-Controlled Study on the Effects of Gotu Kola (Centella Asiatica) on Acoustic Startle Response in Healthy Subjects." *Journal of Clinical Psychopharmacology,* Dec. 2000, 20(6): 680–84.

Shukla, A., A. M. Rasik, and B. N. Dhawan. "Asiaticoside-Induced Elevation of Antioxidant Levels in Healing Wounds." *Phytotherapy Research,* Feb. 1999, 13(1): 50–54.

St. John's Wort

De Vry, J., S. Maurel, R. Schreiber, R. de Beun, and K. R. Jentzsch. "Comparison of Hypericum Extracts with Imipramine and Fluoxetine in Animal Models of Depression and Alcoholism." *European Neuropsychopharmacology,* Dec. 1999, 9(6): 461–68.

Gaster, B., and J. Holroyd. "St John's Wort for Depression: A Systematic Review." *Archives of Internal Medicine,* 24 Jan. 2000, 160(2): 152–56.

Hansgen, K. D., J. Vesper, and M. Ploch. "Multicenter Double-Blind Study Examining the Antidepressant Effectiveness of the Hypericum Extract LI 160." *Journal of Geriatric Psychiatry and Neurology,* Oct. 1994, 7(suppl. 1): S15–18.

Hubner, W. D., S. Lande, and H. Podzuweit. "Hypericum Treatment of Mild Depressions with Somatic Symptoms." *Journal of Geriatric Psychiatry and Neurology,* Oct. 1994, 7(suppl. 1): S12–14.

Kasper S. "Treatment of Seasonal Affective Disorder (SAD) with Hypericum Extract." *Pharmacopsychiatry,* Sept. 1997, 30(suppl. 2): 89–93.

Laakmann, G., C. Schule, T. Baghai, and M. Kieser. "St. John's Wort in Mild to Moderate Depression: The Relevance of Hyperforin for the Clinical Efficacy." *Pharmacopsychiatry,* June 1998, 31(suppl. 1): 54–59.

Linde, K., G. Ramirez, C. D. Mulrow, A. Pauls, W. Weidenhammer, and D. Melchart. "St. John's Wort for Depression: An Overview and Meta-Analysis of Randomised Clinical Trials." *British Medical Journal,* 3 Aug. 1996, 313(7052): 253–58.

Miller, A. L. "St. John's Wort (Hypericum Perforatum): Clinical Effects on Depression and Other Conditions." *Alternative Medicine Review,* Feb. 1998, 3(1): 18–26.

Stevinson, C., and E. Ernst. "Hypericum for Depression: An Update of the Clinical Evidence." *European Neuropsychopharmacology,* Dec. 1999, 9(6): 501–5.

Volz, H. P., and P. Laux. "Potential Treatment for Subthreshold and Mild Depression: A Comparison of St. John's Wort Extracts and Fluoxetine." *Comprehensive Psychiatry,* Mar.–Apr. 2000, 41(2, suppl. 1): 133–37.

5-Hydroxy-Tryptophan (5-HTP)

Birdsall, T. C. "5-Hydroxytryptophan: A Clinically-Effective Serotonin Precursor." *Alternative Medicine Review,* Aug. 1998, 3(4): 271–80.

Byerley, W. F., L. L. Judd, F. W. Reimherr, and B. I. Grosser. "5-Hydroxytryptophan: A Review of Its Antidepressant Efficacy and Adverse Effects." *Journal of Clinical Psychopharmacology,* June 1987, 7(3): 127–37.

Cangiano, C., A. Laviano, M. Del Ben, I. Preziosa, F. Angelico, A. Cascino, and F. Rossi-Fanelli. "Effects of Oral 5-Hydroxy-Tryptophan on Energy Intake and Macronutrient Selection in Non-Insulin-Dependent Diabetic Patients." *International Journal of Obesity and Related Metabolic Disorders,* July 1998, 22(7): 648–54.

De Benedittis, G., and R. Massei. "Serotonin Precursors in Chronic Primary Headache: A Double-Blind Cross-Over Study with L-5-Hydroxytryptophan vs. Placebo." *Journal of Neurosurgical Sciences,* July–Sept. 1985, 29(3): 239–48.

Meyers, S. "Use of Neurotransmitter Precursors for Treatment of Depression." *Alternative Medicine Review,* Feb. 2000, 5(1): 64–71.

D, L-Phenylalanine (DLPA)

Fernstrom, J. D. "Dietary Amino Acids and Brain Function." *Journal of the American Dietetic Association*, Jan. 1994, 94(1): 71–77.

Growdon, J. H., E. L. Cohen, and R. J. Wurtman. "Treatment of Brain Disease with Dietary Precursors of Neurotransmitters." *Annals of Internal Medicine*, Mar. 1977, 86(3): 337–39.

Haze, J. J. "Toward an Understanding of the Rationale for the Use of Dietary Supplementation for Chronic Pain Management: The Serotonin Model." *Cranio: The Journal of Craniomandibular Practice*, Oct. 1991, 9(4): 339–43.

King, R. B. "Pain and Tryptophan." *Journal of Neurosurgery*, July 1980, 53(1): 44–52.

Nurmikko, T., A. Pertovaara, P. J. Pontinen, K. M. Marnela, and S.S. Oja. "Effect of L-Tryptophan Supplementation on Ischemic Pain." *Acupuncture and Electrotherapeutics Research*, 1984, 9(1): 45–55.

Seltzer, S., R. Stoch, R. Marcus, and E. Jackson. "Alteration of Human Pain Thresholds by Nutritional Manipulation and L-Tryptophan Supplementation." *Pain*, Aug. 1982, 13(4): 385–93.

SAM-e

Bottiglieri, T., K. Hyland, and E. H. Reynolds. "The Clinical Potential of Ademetionine (S-Adenosylmethionine) in Neurological Disorders." *Drugs*, Aug. 1994, 48(2): 137–52.

Bottiglieri, T., and K. Hyland. "S-Adenosylmethionine Levels in Psychiatric and Neurological Disorders: A Review." *Acta Neurologica Scandinavia Supplement*, 1994, 154: 19–26.

Bressa, G. M. "S-Adenosyl-L-Methionine (SAM-e) As Antidepressant: Meta-Analysis of Clinical Studies." *Acta Neurologica Scandinavia Supplement*, 1994, 154: 7–14.

Cantoni, G. L., S. H. Mudd, and V. Andreoli. "Affective Disorders and S-Adenosylmethionine: A New Hypothesis." *Trends in Neuroscience*, Sept. 1989, 12(9): 319–24.

Rosenbaum, J. F., M. Fava, W. E. Falk, M. H. Pollack, L. S. Cohen, B. M. Cohen, and G. S. Zubenko. "The Antidepressant Potential of Oral

S-Adenosyl-L-Methionine." *Acta Psychiatrica Scandinavia*, May 1990, 81(5): 432–36.

Salmaggi, P., G. M. Bressa, G. Nicchia, M. Coniglio, P. La Greca, and C. Le Grazie. "Double-Blind, Placebo-Controlled Study of S-Adenosyl-L-Methionine in Depressed Postmenopausal Women." *Psychotherapy and Psychosomatics*, 1993, 59(1): 34 40.

Chapter 11: Metabolic-Support Supplements (Blood-Sugar Control, Muscle Maintenance, and Immune Enhancement)

Chromium

Anderson, R. A. "Effects of Chromium on Body Composition and Weight Loss." *Nutrition Review*, Sept. 1998, 56(9): 266–70.

McCarty, M. F. "Chromium and Other Insulin Sensitizers May Enhance Glucagon Secretion: Implications for Hypoglycemia and Weight Control." *Medical Hypotheses*, Feb. 1996, 46(2): 77–80.

Trent, L. K., and D. Thieding-Cancel. "Effects of Chromium Picolinate on Body Composition." *Journal of Sports Medicine and Physical Fitness*, Dec. 1995, 35(4): 273–80.

Uusitupa, M. I., L. Mykkanen, O. Siitonen, M. Laakso, H. Sarlund, P. Kolehmainen, T. Rasanen, J. Kumpulainen, and K. Pyorala. "Chromium Supplementation in Impaired Glucose Tolerance of Elderly: Effects on Blood Glucose, Plasma Insulin, C-Peptide and Lipid Levels." *British Journal of Nutrition*, July 1992, 68(1): 209–16.

Vanadium

Cohen, N., M. Halberstam, P. Shlimovich, C. J. Chang, H. Shamoon, and L. Rossetti. "Oral Vanadyl Sulfate Improves Hepatic and Peripheral Insulin Sensitivity in Patients with Non-Insulin-Dependent Diabetes Mellitus." *Journal of Clinical Investigations*, June 1995, 95(6): 2501–9.

Goldfine, A. B., M. E. Patti, L. Zuberi, B. J. Goldstein, R. LeBlanc, E. J. Landaker, Z. Y. Jiang, G. R. Willsky, and C. R. Kahn. "Metabolic Effects of Vanadyl Sulfate in Humans with Non-Insulin-Dependent Diabetes Mellitus: In Vivo and In Vitro Studies." *Metabolism*, Mar. 2000, 49(3): 400–10.

Jandhyala, B. S., and G. J. Hom. "Minireview: Physiological and Pharmacological Properties of Vanadium." *Life Science*, 3 Oct. 1983, 33(14): 1325–40.

Preuss, H. G., S. T. Jarrell, R. Scheckenbach, S. Lieberman, and R. A. Anderson. "Comparative Effects of Chromium, Vanadium and Gymnema Sylvestre on Sugar-Induced Blood Pressure Elevations in SHR." *Journal of the American College of Nutrition*, Apr. 1998, 17(2): 116–23.

Banaba Leaf

Kakuda, T., I. Sakane, T. Takihara, Y. Ozaki, H. Takeuchi, and M. Kuroyanagi. "Hypoglycemic Effect of Extracts from Lagerstroemia Speciosa L. Leaves in Genetically Diabetic KK-AY Mice." *Bioscience, Biotechnology, Biochemistry*, Feb. 1996, 60(2): 204–8.

Suzuki, Y., T. Unno, M. Ushitani, K. Hayashi, and T. Kakuda. "Antiobesity Activity of Extracts from Lagerstroemia Speciosa L. Leaves on Female KK-AY Mice." *Journal of Nutrition Science and Vitaminology.* Tokyo, Dec. 1999, 45(6): 791–95.

Gymnema

Baskaran, K., B. Kizar Ahamath, K. Radha Shanmugasundaram, and E. R. Shanmugasundaram. "Antidiabetic Effect of a Leaf Extract from Gymnema Sylvestre in Non-Insulin-Dependent Diabetes Mellitus Patients." *Journal of Ethnopharmacology*, Oct. 1990, 30(3): 295–300.

Shanmugasundaram, E. R., G. Rajeswari, K. Baskaran, B. R. Rajesh Kumar, K. Radha Shanmugasundaram, B. Kizar Ahmath. "Use of Gymnema Sylvestre Leaf Extract in the Control of Blood Glucose in Insulin-Dependent Diabetes Mellitus." *Journal of Ethnopharmacology*, Oct. 1990, 30(3): 281–94.

Shanmugasundaram, K. R., C. Panneerselvam, P. Samudram, and E. R. Shanmugasundaram. "The Insulinotropic Activity of Gymnema Sylvestre, R. Br., an Indian Medical Herb Used in Controlling Diabetes Mellitus." *Pharmacological Research Communications*, May 1981, 13(5): 475–86.

Shimizu, K., A. Iino, J. Nakajima, K. Tanaka, S. Nakajyo, N. Urakawa, M. Atsuchi, T. Wada, and C. Yamashita. "Suppression of Glucose Absorption by Some Fractions Extracted from Gymnema Sylvestre

Leaves." *Journal of Veterinary Medicine and Science*, Apr. 1997, 59(4): 245–51.

DHEA (Dehydroepiandrosterone)

Brown, G. A., M. D. Vukovich, R. L. Sharp, T. A. Reifenrath, K. A. Parsons, and D. S. King. "Effect of Oral DHEA on Serum Testosterone and Adaptations to Resistance Training in Young Men." *Journal of Applied Physiology*, Dec. 1999, 87(6): 2274–83.

Filaire, E., P. Duche, and G. Lac. "Effects of Amount of Training on the Saliva Concentrations of Cortisol, Dehydroepiandrosterone and on the Dehydroepiandrosterone: Cortisol Concentration Ratio in Women over 16 Weeks of Training." *European Journal of Applied Physiology and Occupational Physiology*, Oct. 1998, 78(5): 466–71.

Filaire, E., P. Duche, and G. Lac. "Effects of Training for Two Ball Games on the Saliva Response of Adrenocortical Hormones to Exercise in Elite Sportswomen." *European Journal of Applied Physiology and Occupational Physiology*, Apr. 1998, 77(5): 452–56.

Keizer, H., G. M. Janssen, P. Menheere, and G. Kranenburg. "Changes in Basal Plasma Testosterone, Cortisol, and Dehydroepiandrosterone Sulfate in Previously Untrained Males and Females Preparing for a Marathon." *International Journal of Sports Medicine*, Oct. 1989, 10(suppl. 3): S139–45.

Zinc

Abbasi, A. A., A. S. Prasad, P. Rabbani, and E. DuMouchelle. "Experimental Zinc Deficiency in Man: Effect on Testicular Function." *Journal of Laboratory and Clinical Medicine*, Sept. 1980, 96(3): 544–50.

Lukaski, H. C. "Magnesium, Zinc, and Chromium Nutriture and Physical Activity." *American Journal of Clinical Nutrition*, Aug. 2000, 72(2, suppl.): S585–93.

McDonald, R., and C. L. Keen. "Iron, Zinc and Magnesium Nutrition and Athletic Performance." *Sports Medicine*, Mar. 1988, 5(3): 171–84.

Nishi Y. "Anemia and Zinc Deficiency in the Athlete." *Journal of the American College of Nutrition*, Aug. 1996, 15(4): 323–24.

Prasad, A. S. "Zinc Deficiency in Human Subjects." *Progress in Clinical and Biological Research*, 1983, 129: 1–33.

Cordyceps

Bao, T. T., G. F. Wang, and Y. L. Yang. "Pharmacological Actions of Cordyceps Sinensis." *Chung Hsi I Chieh Ho Tsa Chih,* June 1988, 8(6): 352-54, 325–26.

Kuo, Y. C., W. J. Tsai, M. S. Shiao, C. F. Chen, and C. Y. Lin. "Cordyceps Sinensis as an Immunomodulatory Agent." *American Journal of Chinese Medicine,* 1996, 24(2): 111–25.

Zhu, J. S., G. M. Halpern, and K. Jones. "The Scientific Rediscovery of an Ancient Chinese Herbal Medicine: Cordyceps Sinensis: Part I." *Journal of Alternative and Complementary Medicine,* Fall 1998, 4(3): 289–303.

Zhu, J. S., G. M. Halpern, and K. Jones. "The Scientific Rediscovery of a Precious Ancient Chinese Herbal Regimen: Cordyceps Sinensis: Part II." *Journal of Alternative and Complementary Medicine,* Winter 1998, 4(4): 429–57.

Conjugated Linoleic Acid (CLA)

Stangl, G. I. "Conjugated Linoleic Acids Exhibit a Strong Fat-to-Lean Partitioning Effect, Reduce Serum VLDL Lipids and Redistribute Tissue Lipids in Food-Restricted Rats." *Journal of Nutrition,* May 2000, 130(5): 1140–46.

Zambell, K. L., N. L. Keim, M. D. Van Loan, B. Gale, P. Benito, D. S. Kelley, and G. J. Nelson. "Conjugated Linoleic Acid Supplementation in Humans: Effects on Body Composition and Energy Expenditure." *Lipids,* July 2000, 35(7): 777–82.

HMB (Hydroxy-Methyl-Butyrate)

Kreider, R. B., M. Ferreira, M. Wilson, and A. L. Almada. "Effects of Calcium Beta-Hydroxy-Beta-Methylbutyrate (HMB) Supplementation During Resistance-Training on Markers of Catabolism, Body Composition and Strength." *International Journal of Sports Medicine,* Nov. 1999, 20(8): 503–9.

Nissen, S., R. Sharp, M. Ray, J. A. Rathmacher, D. Rice, J. C. Fuller, Jr., A. S. Connelly, and N. Abumrad. "Effect of Leucine Metabolite Beta-Hydroxy-Beta-Methylbutyrate on Muscle Metabolism During Resistance-Exercise Training." *Journal of Applied Physiology,* Nov. 1996, 81(5): 2095–104.

Panton, L. B., J. A. Rathmacher, S. Baier, and S. Nissen. "Nutritional Supplementation of the Leucine Metabolite Beta-Hydroxy-Beta-Methylbutyrate (HMB) During Resistance Training." *Nutrition*, Sept. 2000, 16(9): 734–39.

Slater, G. J., and D. Jenkins. "Beta-Hydroxy-Beta-Methylbutyrate (HMB) Supplementation and the Promotion of Muscle Growth and Strength." *Sports Medicine*, Aug. 2000, 30(2): 105–16.

Echinacea

Abdullah, T. "A Strategic Call to Utilize Echinacea-Garlic in Flu-Cold Seasons." *Journal of the Natural Medicine Association*, Jan. 2000, 92(1): 48–51.

Giles, J. T., C. T. Palat 3rd, S. H. Chien, Z. G. Chang, and D. T. Kennedy. "Evaluation of Echinacea for Treatment of the Common Cold." *Pharmacotherapy*, June 2000, 20(6): 690–97.

Gunning, K. "Echinacea in the Treatment and Prevention of Upper Respiratory Tract Infections." *Western Journal of Medicine*, Sept. 1999, 171(3): 198–200.

Lindenmuth, G. F., and E. B. Lindenmuth. "The Efficacy of Echinacea Compound Herbal Tea Preparation on the Severity and Duration of Upper Respiratory and Flu Symptoms: A Randomized, Double-Blind Placebo-Controlled Study." *Journal of Alternative and Complementary Medicine*, Aug. 2000, 6(4): 327–34.

Goldenseal

"Berberine." *Alternative Medicine Review*, Apr. 2000, 5(2): 175–77.

Blecher, M. B., and K. Douglass. "Gold in Goldenseal." *Hospital Health Network*, 20 Oct. 1997, 71(20): 50–52.

Iwasa, K., M. Moriyasu, and B. Nader. "Fungicidal and Herbicidal Activities of Berberine-Related Alkaloids." *Bioscience, Biotechnology, and Biochemistry*, Sept. 2000, 64(9): 1998–2000.

Asian Mushrooms

Borchers, A. T., J. S. Stern, R. M. Hackman, C. L. Keen, and M. E. Gershwin. "Mushrooms, Tumors, and Immunity." *Proceedings of the Society for Experimental Biology and Medicine*, Sept. 1999, 221(4): 281–93.

Chang R. "Functional Properties of Edible Mushrooms." *Nutrition Review*, Nov. 1996, 54(11, pt. 2): S91–93.

Kidd, P. M. "The Use of Mushroom Glucans and Proteoglycans in Cancer Treatment." *Alternative Medicine Review*, Feb. 2000, 5(1): 4–27.

Ooi, V. E., and F. Liu. "Immunomodulation and Anti-Cancer Activity of Polysaccharide-Protein Complexes." *Current Medicinal Chemistry*, July 2000, 7(7): 715–29.

Probiotics/Prebiotics

Alles, M. S., J. G. Hautvast, F. M. Nagengast, R. Hartemink, K. M. Van Laere, and J. B. Jansen. "Fate of Fructo-Oligosaccharides in the Human Intestine." *British Journal of Nutrition*, Aug. 1996, 76(2): 211–21.

Arunachalam, K., H. S. Gill, and R. K. Chandra. "Enhancement of Natural Immune Function by Dietary Consumption of Bifidobacterium Lactis (HN019)." *European Journal of Clinical Nutrition*, Mar. 2000, 54(3): 263–67.

Bouhnik, Y., B. Flourie, M. Riottot, N. Bisetti, M. F. Gailing, A. Guibert, F. Bornet, and J. C. Rambaud. "Effects of Fructo-Oligosaccharides Ingestion on Fecal Bifidobacteria and Selected Metabolic Indexes of Colon Carcinogenesis in Healthy Humans." *Nutrition and Cancer*, 1996, 26(1): 21–9.

Brady, L. J., D. D. Gallaher, and F. F. Busta. "The Role of Probiotic Cultures in the Prevention of Colon Cancer." *Journal of Nutrition*, Feb. 2000, 130(2, suppl.): S410–14.

Collins, M. D., and G. R. Gibson. "Probiotics, Prebiotics, and Synbiotics: Approaches for Modulating the Microbial Ecology of the Gut." *American Journal of Clinical Nutrition*, May 1999, 69(5): S1052–57.

Cunningham-Rundles, S., S. Ahrne, S. Bengmark, R. Johann-Liang, F. Marshall, L. Metakis, C. Califano, A. M. Dunn, C. Grassey, G. Hinds, and J. Cervia. "Probiotics and Immune Response." *American Journal of Gastroenterology*, Jan. 2000, 95(1, suppl.): S22–25.

Dugas, B., A. Mercenier, I. Lenoir-Wijnkoop, C. Arnaud, N. Dugas, and E. Postaire. "Immunity and Probiotics." *Immunology Today*, Sept. 1999, 20(9): 387–90.

Goldin, B. R. "Health Benefits of Probiotics." *British Journal of Nutrition*, Oct. 1998, 80(4): S203-7.

Hirayama, K., and J. Rafter. "The Role of Probiotic Bacteria in Cancer Prevention." *Microbes and Infection*, May 2000, 2(6): 681-86.

Bioflavonoids

Bravo, L. "Polyphenols: Chemistry, Dietary Sources, Metabolism, and Nutritional Significance." *Nutrition Review*, Nov. 1998, 56(11): 317–33.

Damianaki, A., E. Bakogeorgou, M. Kampa, G. Notas, A. Hatzoglou, S. Panagiotou, C. Gemetzi, E. Kouroumalis, P. M. Martin, and E. Castanas. "Potent Inhibitory Action of Red Wine Polyphenols on Human Breast Cancer Cells." *Journal of Cellular Biochemistry*, 6 June 2000, 78(3): 429–41.

Goldbohm, R. A., M. G. Hertog, H. A. Brants, G. van Poppel, and P. A. van den Brandt. "Consumption of Black Tea and Cancer Risk: A Prospective Cohort Study." *Journal of the National Cancer Institute*, 17 Jan. 1996, 88(2): 93–100.

Kuo, S. M. "Dietary Flavonoid and Cancer Prevention: Evidence and Potential Mechanism." *Critical Reviews in Oncology*, 1997, 8(1): 47–69.

Vitamin A

Daudu, P. A., D. S. Kelley, P. C. Taylor, B. J. Burri, and M. M. Wu. "Effect of a Low Beta-Carotene Diet on the Immune Functions of Adult Women." *American Journal of Clinical Nutrition*, Dec. 1994, 60(6): 969–72.

Fortes, C., F. Forastiere, N. Agabiti, V. Fano, R. Pacifici, F. Virgili, G. Piras, L. Guidi, C. Bartoloni, A. Tricerri, P. Zuccaro, S. Ebrahim, and C. A. Perucci. "The Effect of Zinc and Vitamin A Supplementation on Immune Response in an Older Population." *Journal of the American Geriatric Society*, Jan. 1998, 46(1): 19–26.

Rumore, M. M. "Vitamin A as an Immunomodulating Agent." *Clinical Pharmacology*, July 1993, 12(7): 506–14.

Semba, R. D. "Vitamin A and Immunity to Viral, Bacterial and Protozoan Infections." *Proceedings of the Nutrition Society*, Aug. 1999, 58(3): 719–27.

West, C. E., J. H. Rombout, A. J. van der Zijpp, and S. R. Sijtsma. "Vitamin A and Immune Function." *Proceedings of the Nutrition Society*, Aug. 1991, 50(2): 251–62.

Selenium

Comstock, G. W., A. J. Alberg, H. Y. Huang, K. Wu, A. E. Burke, S. C. Hoffman, E. P. Norkus, M. Gross, R. G. Cutler, J. S. Morris, V. L. Spate, and H. J. Helzlsouer. "The Risk of Developing Lung Cancer Associated with Antioxidants in the Blood: Ascorbic Acid, Carotenoids, Alpha-Tocopherol, Selenium, and Total Peroxyl Radical Absorbing Capacity." *Cancer Epidemiology, Biomarkers, and Prevention*, Nov. 1997, 6(11): 907–16.

Dorgan, J. F., and A. Schatzkin. "Antioxidant Micronutrients in Cancer Prevention." *Hematologic Oncology Clinics of North America*, Feb. 1991, 5(1): 43–68.

Lamberg L. "Diet May Affect Skin Cancer Prevention." *Journal of the American Medical Association*, 13 May 1998, 279(18): 1427–28.

Resources

Numerous excellent resources are available on the topics of relaxation and other stress-management techniques, as well as exercise, diet, and supplements. A few of them are listed here.

Stress Management and Avoidance

Don't Sweat the Small Stuff ... and It's All Small Stuff, by Richard Carlson (Hyperion, 1997).

Fight Fat after Forty, by Pamela Peeke (Penguin, 2001).

Simplify Your Life, by Elaine St. James (Hyperion, 1994).

Why Zebras Don't Get Ulcers, by Robert M. Sapolsky (W. H. Freeman and Co., 1998).

You Can Choose to Be Happy, by Tom G. Stevens (Wheeler Sutton, 1998).

Exercise

Body for Life: Twelve Weeks to Mental and Physical Strength, by Bill Phillips and Michael D'Orso (HarperCollins, 1999).

When Working Out Isn't Working Out, by Michael Gerrish (Griffin Trade Paperback, 1999).

Nutrition

Eat, Drink, and Be Healthy: The Harvard Medical School Guide to Healthy Eating, by Walter Willett, P. J. Skerrett, and Edward L. Giovannucci (Simon and Schuster, 2001).

Fad-Free Nutrition, by Frederick Stare and Elizabeth Whelan (Hunter House, 1998).

Strong Women Eat Well: Nutritional Strategies for a Healthy Body and Mind, by Miriam E. Nelson and Judy Knipe (Putnam, 2001).

The Zone: Dietary Road Map to Losing Weight Permanently, by Barry Sears and Bill Lawren (HarperCollins, 1995).

Supplements

Chinese Herbal Medicine Made Easy: Effective and Natural Remedies for Common Illnesses, by Thomas Richard Joiner (Hunter House, 2001).

Magic Bullets or Modern Snake Oil? Your Guide to Understanding Dietary Supplements, by Shawn M. Talbott (Haworth Press, forthcoming 2002).

SupplementWatch website: www.SupplementWatch.com. (Note: Shawn M. Talbott was one of the original founders of Supplement-Watch.com and has contributed extensively to the website. Readers may notice some overlap between the contents of certain supplement descriptions on the website and those in this book.)

INDEX

A

adaptogens, 145–154, 203–204; ashwagandha (*Withania somnifera*), 94, 148–149; astragalus, 152–154; ginseng, 146–148; rhodiola (*Rhodiola rosea/Rhodiola crenulata*), 151–152; schisandra (*Schisandra chinensis*), 150–151; suma (*Pfaffia paniculata*), 149–150
Addison's disease, 7–8, 24
adrenal glands, 22–24
aging, *xiv*, 72–76; and memory loss, 68–69; and weight gain, 41–42, 44
alcohol, 86
Alzheimer's disease, 64, 68–69, 140
American College of Nutrition, 96
American Dietetic Association, 96
American Nutraceutical Association, 96
anticatabolics (muscle maintainers), 177–181

antidepressants. *See* supplements, antidepressant
antioxidants, 118; and the common cold, 119
anxiety, 64–67, 157. *See also* supplements, antianxiety
Arctic root. *See* rhodiola
ashwagandha (*Withania somnifera*), 94, 148–149
astragalus, 152–154
autoimmune disease, 57–61

B

banaba leaf (*Lagestroemia speciosa*), 173–175
B-complex vitamins, 93, 96–97, 114, 125–127
berberine, 184
Bifidobacteria bifidum, 185
bioflavonoids, 186
bitter orange. *See* synephrine
blood sugar, 171–176, 204–207
brain waves, 51, 131–133
branched-chain amino acids (BCAAs), 142–144
Brazilian ginseng. *See* suma

THE ART OF GETTING WELL: A Five-Step Plan for Maximizing Health When You Have a Chronic Illness
by David Spero, R.N., Foreword by Martin L. Rossman, M.D.

Self-management programs have become a key way for people to deal with chronic illness. In this book, David Spero brings together the medical, psychological, and spiritual aspects of getting well in a five-step approach that asks you to slow down and use your energy for the things and people that matter; make small, progressive changes that build self-confidence; get help and nourish the social ties that are crucial for well-being; value your body and treat it with affection and respect; and take responsibility for getting the best care and health you can.

224 pages ... Paperback $15.95 ... Hardcover $25.95

CHINESE HERBAL MEDICINE MADE EASY: Natural and Effective Remedies for Common Illnesses
by Thomas Richard Joiner

Chinese herbal medicine is an ancient system for maintaining health and prolonging life. This book demystifies the subject, by providing clear explanations and easy-to-read alphabetical listings of more than 750 herbal remedies for over 250 common illnesses ranging from acid reflux and AIDS to breast cancer, pain management, sexual dysfunction, and weight loss. Whether you are a newcomer to herbology or a seasoned practitioner, you will find this book to be a valuable addition to your health library.

432 pages ... Paperback $24.95 ... Hardcover $34.95

FAD-FREE NUTRITION
by Frederick J. Stare, M.D., Ph.D., and Elizabeth M. Whelan, Sc.D., MPH

From the American Council on Science and Health, a no-nonsense book that challenges trendy diets and offers sound information on how to eat normally and eat right. From explaining why the produce at the supermarket is indeed safe, to describing which foods can boost immune system functioning, to showing how easy the food pyramid really is to understand and follow, this book puts the joy back into food.

256 pages ... Paperback $14.95